Psychiatry in Europe

Edited by

TOM SENSKY
CORNELIUS KATONA
STUART MONTGOMERY

Psychiatry in Europe

Directions and Developments

GASKELL

Gaskell is an imprint of the Royal College of Psychiatrists,
17 Belgrave Square, London SW1

British Library Cataloguing-in-Publication Data
Psychiatry in Europe: Directions and Developments
  I. Sensky, Tom
  616.890094

ISBN 0-902241-71-0

Distributed in North America
by American Psychiatric Press, Inc.
ISBN 0-88048-635-X

Publication of this book was made possible by the
kind assistance of Glaxo Pharmaceuticals.

Phototypeset by Dobbie Typesetting Limited, Tavistock, Devon
Printed by Henry Ling Ltd, The Dorset Press, Dorchester, Dorset

Contents

v

Part IV. Psychological interventions

Part V. Service delivery

Part VI. Attitudes to mental illness

Contributors

Gerd Baumann, PhD, FRAI, Reader in Anthropology, Research Centre of Religion and Society, University of Amsterdam, Rokin 84, NL 1012 KX Amsterdam, The Netherlands

Douglas H. R. Blackwood, PhD, FRCP, FRCPsych, Reader in Psychiatry, University of Edinburgh Department of Psychiatry, Royal Edinburgh Hospital, Morningside Park, Edinburgh

Mark Bourgeois, MD, PhD, Professor, Centre Hospitalo-Universitaire de Bordeaux, Centre Carreire, 121 rue de la Béchade, 33076 Bordeaux Cédex, France

Ian F. Brockington, MD, FRCP, FRCPsych, Professor of Psychiatry, University of Birmingham, Queen Elizabeth Psychiatric Hospital, Birmingham B15 2TH

Tim Bullock, MBBS, Lecturer in Psychiatry, St Mary's Hospital Medical School, Norfolk Place, London W2 1PG

Vincent F. Caillard, MD, Centre Esquirol, CHRU de Caen, 14033 Caen, France

Jean Cottraux, MD, PhD, Consultant Psychiatrist, Department of Psychiatry and Medical Psychology, Hôpital Neurologique, 59 Boulevard Pinel 69394, Lyon, France

Francis Creed, MD, FRCP, FRCPsych, Professor of Community Psychiatry, Department of Psychiatry, University of Manchester, Oxford Road, Manchester M13 9WL

Hilton Davis, BA, DipClinPsych, CPsychol, FBPsS, PhD, Reader in Psychology, Child Mental Health Services, Bloomfield Clinic, Guy's Hospital, St Thomas Street, London SE1 9RT

Valsamma Eapen, MBBS, MRCPsych, Lecturer in Child Psychiatry, Academic Department of Psychiatry, University College Medical School, Middlesex Hospital, Mortimer Street, London W1N 8AA

Martin Eisemann, MD, Associate Professor of Psychiatry, University of Umeå, Umeå, Sweden

Anne E. Farmer, MD, FRCPsych, DPM, Senior Lecturer, Department of Psychological Medicine, University of Wales College of Medicine, Heath Park, Cardiff CF4 4XN

Naomi Fineberg, MA, MRCPsych, Senior Registrar in Psychiatry, St Mary's Hospital Medical School, Norfolk Place, London W2 1PG

Paloma Galdos, MD, Registrar, Centre Hospitalo-Universitaire de Bordeaux, Centre Carreire, 121 rue de la Béchade, 33076 Bordeaux Cédex, France

Daniel Gérard, Resident, Centre d'Exploration et de Recherche Médicales par Emission de Positons (CERMEP), Hôpital Neurologique, 59 Boulevard Pinel 69394, Lyon, France

Robert Giel, Professor of Social Psychiatry, Department of Social Psychiatry, University of Groningen, Academisch Ziekenhuis Groningen, PO Box 30.001, 9700 RB Groningen, The Netherlands

Peter Hall, MBBS, PhD, FRCPsych, DPM, Medical Director, The Woodbourne Clinic, 21 Woodbourne Road, Birmingham B17 8BY

Thomas Herzog, DrMed, DiplPsych, Vice-Chairman, Abteilung Psychotherapie und Psychosomatische Medizin der Universität Freiburg, Hauptstrasse 8, 79104 Freiburg, Germany

Frits Huyse, MD, PhD, Associate Professor, Department of Psychiatry, Vrije Universiteit Amsterdam, De Boelelaan 1117, PO Box 7075, NL-1107 MB Amsterdam, The Netherlands

Cornelius L. E. Katona, Professor of Psychiatry of the Elderly, University College Medical School, Middlesex Hospital, Mortimer Street, London W1N 8AA

Michael Langenbach, MD, Department of Psychosomatic Medicine and Psychotherapy, Heinrich Heine University, Dusseldorf, Germany

Herman Kluiter, Senior Research Psychologist, Department of Social Psychiatry, University of Groningen, Academisch Ziekenhuis Groningen, PO Box 30.001, 9700 RB Groningen, The Netherlands

Glyn Lewis, MRCPsych, PhD, Senior Lecturer, Department of Epidemiology and General Practice, Institute of Psychiatry, De Crespigny Park, London SE5 8AF, and London School of Hygiene and Tropical Medicine, Keppel Street, London WC1

Antonio Lobo, MD, PhD, Professor of Psychiatry, Universidad de Zaragoza, Departamento de Psiquiatria, Hospital Clinico Universitario, Planta 11, E-50009 Zaragoza, Spain

Michael Madianos, MD, Associate Professor of Psychiatry, University of Athens, Athens, Greece

Andrea L. Malizia, Wellcome Training Fellow, MRC Cyclotron Unit, Hammersmith Hospital, DuCane Road, London W12 0HS

Ulrik F. Malt, MD, Professor of Psychiatry, Department of Psychosomatic and Behavioural Medicine, Universitet Oslo, Rikshospitalet, Psykosomatisk avdeling, Pilestredet 32, N-0027 Oslo 1, Norway

Anthony Mann, MD, MPhil, FRCP, FRCPsych, Professor, Department of Epidemiology and General Practice, Institute of Psychiatry, De Crespigny Park, London SE5 8AF

Stuart A. Montgomery, MD, FRCPsych, Professor of Psychiatry, St Mary's Hospital Medical School, Norfolk Place, London W2 1PG

Walter J. Muir, MRCPsych, MRC Clinical Scientist, University of Edinburgh Department of Psychiatry, Royal Edinburgh Hospital, Morningside Park, Edinburgh

Gerhardt Nissen, MD, Emeritus Professor of Child and Adolescent Psychiatry, Bayerische Julius-Maximilians University, Füchsleinstrasse 15, Würzburg, 97080 Germany

William Ll. Parry-Jones, MA, MD, FRCP, FRCPsych, Professor of Child and Adolescent Psychiatry, University of Glasgow, Royal Hospital for Sick Children, Glasgow G3 8SJ

Pierre Pichot, Honorary Professor of Psychiatry, University of Paris, and Membre de l'Académie Nationale de Médecine, 24 rue des Fossés-Saint-Jacques, F-75005, Paris, France

Ann Roberts, MA, MRCPsych, Senior Registrar, St Mary's Hospital Medical School, Norfolk Place, London W2 1PG

Mary M. Robertson, MBChB, MD, DPM, FRCPsych, Senior Lecturer in Psychiatry, Academic Department of Psychiatry, University College Medical School, Middlesex Hospital, Mortimer Street, London W1N 8AA

Paloma Ruiz, MD, formerly Senior House Officer, Department of Psychiatry, University Hospital, Nottingham NG7 2UH

Tom Sensky, BSc, PhD, MB, FRCPsych, Senior Lecturer in Psychiatry, Charing Cross and Westminster Medical School, West Middlesex University Hospital, Isleworth, Middlesex TW7 6AF

Andrew Sims, MA, MD, FRCPsych, FRCP(Ed), Professor of Psychiatry, St James's University Hospital, Leeds LS9 7TF

Barbara Stein, DiplPsych, Clinical Research Psychologist, Abteilung Psychotherapie und Psychosomatische Medizin der Universität Freiburg, Hauptstrasse 8, 79104 Freiburg, Germany

Vlassis Tomaras, MD, Assistant Professor of Psychiatry, University of Athens, Eginition Hospital, 74 Vas. Sofias Avenue, Athens 115 28, Greece

Jim van Os, MSc, MRCPsych, Lecturer and MRC Training Fellow, Department of Psychological Medicine, Institute of Psychiatry, De Crespigny Park, London SE5 8AF

Agnes Vetró, MD, PhD, Associate Professor of Child and Adolescent Psychiatry, Department of Pediatrics, Albert Szent-Györgyi Medical University, Szeged, 6725 Hungary

Andreas Warnke, MD, Professor of Child and Adolescent Psychiatry, Bayerische Julius-Maximilians University, Füchsleinstrasse 15, Würzburg, 97080 Germany

Lucia Whitney, MD, Senior Registrar in Child and Adolescent Psychiatry, Thorneywood Unit, Nottingham NG3 6LF.

Durk Wiersma, Associate Professor, Department of Social Psychiatry, University of Groningen, Academisch Ziekenhuis Groningen, PO Box 30.001, 9700 RB Groningen, The Netherlands

Julie Williams, PhD, Lecturer, Department of Psychological Medicine, University of Wales College of Medicine, Heath Park, Cardiff CF4 4XN

Foreword

In looking for an obvious bridge between the two major areas of the world where psychiatric research and creativity have flourished, Europe and North America, one would necessarily alight upon the British Isles. We, on these islands, have our cultural and historical roots in European psychiatry, and our present style of practice is similar to that of some European countries. Meanwhile, our language we hold in common (almost) with North America, and for the last few decades there has been much greater exchange of personnel with Canada and the United States of America than with Europe. British medicine has a lot to learn from, and contribute to, research, theory and practice in continental Europe, although our geographical isolation and temperamental aloofness has to some extent prevented this until recently.

With this background, it was with great pleasure and anticipation that we, many British psychiatrists and a good number from many different European countries, attended the Autumn Quarterly Meeting of the Royal College of Psychiatrists, ''Psychiatry in Europe'' in October 1992 at the National Exhibition Centre, and most appropriately, right beside Birmingham International Airport. We were not disappointed; it was an excellent programme and the meeting was a considerable success.

The chapters of this book are some of the papers, fully revised, of that symposium, and they represent just a few of the areas where dialogue between continental European and British psychiatry has been profitable. Part VI of this book, ''Attitudes to mental illness'', shows how enormously these vary in each European country. Attitudes to psychiatry, and the psychiatrists, differ hugely from tolerance to fear, from breathless admiration to ribald disrespect; if one moves outside Europe to south-east Asia or to Africa, beliefs and opinions concerning mental illness are even more varied.

''Service delivery'' (Part V) is a practical topic where we really can do each other a lot of good, by comparing notes and finding out what worked well for other people, and why. Is the move towards community care a logical extension of the humane approaches to treatment inherited from the last century, or a Gadarene leap over the precipice into the unknown? How do we differ in our use of legal detention, compulsory treatment, or restraint? How can we best serve our medical colleagues in meeting the needs of their patients, both physical and mental?

There are surprisingly large differences between European countries in the manner in which knowledge of psychology has penetrated psychiatric practice; even the word psychology appears to have somewhat different nuances in different European languages. The section on this topic (Part IV) makes a start in comparing different approaches. It is a huge subject and will merit much future consideration.

There have been many advances in biological psychiatry in recent years, both in understanding the basic pathophysiology, and in treatment. Such work will be greatly facilitated by communicating the findings of this research and discussing methods and techniques with collaborators from other European countries. We are much more likely to make further progress if we adhere to rational nosology and the basic principles of descriptive psychopathology (Parts I–III).

Psychiatry in Europe: Directions and Developments is an intriguing beginning to what one hopes will be increasingly creative contact between all European psychiatrists. There was much fruitful cross-fertilisation in the past in understanding mental illnesses and developing effective methods of treatment between psychiatrists in continental Europe and those in Britain. In the more recent past this contact seemed to have diminished, while much closer links were established between the United Kingdom and Ireland with psychiatry in North America. It is high time for the balance to be redressed and this book is commended to the reader as a valuable contribution to help us all, as European psychiatrists, to understand and learn from each other.

Andrew Sims
Immediate Past President,
Royal College of Psychiatrists

Introduction

The chapters of this book all review recent advances or innovative developments in psychiatry. Common to all the contributions is their pertinence to current psychiatry in Europe. Some chapters describe direct comparisons between different European countries. Examples are the chapter by Whitney and colleagues on legal detention of psychiatric patients, and those by Hall and colleagues, and Van Os and colleagues on attitudes to psychiatry and mental illness. Other contributors were asked to review important topics which are widely applicable across countries and cultures, ranging from family interventions in schizophrenia (Tomaras), to biological markers in the major psychoses (Blackwood & Muir). Another group of chapters, exemplified by the account by Herzog and colleagues of psychosomatic medical practice and Davis' description of counselling support for families of disabled children, describe innovative models of practice which offer lessons for psychiatry beyond their own practice or country of origin. We are particularly fortunate to be able to include the full text of Professor Pierre Pichot's 1992 Maudsley Lecture.

The contributors were among those who presented papers at the scientific meeting of the Royal College of Psychiatrists in Birmingham in October 1992. This meeting had a strongly pan-European emphasis, with participants and invited speakers from many European countries. The contributors were chosen in part by popular demand based on favourable comments about their presentations. Each was invited to provide an updated review based on the topic of the original paper. Although not intended to represent a comprehensive account of the proceedings of the Birmingham meeting, the chapters of the book together cover a wide range of topics.

The contributions hold something of value for all those with an interest in modern psychiatry. Readers, whether career psychiatrists, psychiatric trainees, or others, have the opportunity to review recent developments, particularly from Europe, in aspects of psychiatry with which they may be familiar, as well as learning something about less familiar and innovative topics. Just as the *Psychiatry in Europe* meeting gave participants the opportunity to broaden their horizons geographically as well as professionally, we hope that this book might have a similar influence on its readers.

Tom Sensky

Part I. Phenomenology

1 Nosological models in psychiatry

PIERRE PICHOT

The botanical classifications

"Nature, in the production of diseases, is uniform and consistent; so much so, that for the same disease in different persons the symptoms are for the most part the same; and the self-same phenomena that you could observe in the sickness of a Socrates you would observe in the sickness of a simpleton. Just so the universal characters of a plant are extending to every individual of the species; and whoever (I speak in the way of illustration) should accurately describe the colour, the taste, the smell, the figure, etc. of the single violet would find that his description held good, there or thereabout, for all the violets of that particular species upon the face of the earth."

This statement, written at the end of the 17th century by Thomas Sydenham (1682), marks the birth of the modern history of nosology. From then on disease became a composite term describing the common features of a variety of individual cases, and nosology a branch of medicine concerned with their definition, while nosography dealt with the hierarchical distribution of those entities: species classified into classes, orders, and genders.

During the 18th century classification reached its golden age in the domain of natural sciences. Those in this age of enlightenment were convinced that Nature submitted to the rules of reason and that it was possible by rational methods to unravel its constituting elements and their organisation. Those were the ideas of the chemists, such as Cavendish, Priestley, Scheele, and Lavoisier, and, of the botanists. Carl von Linnaeus (Linné) through his publication of the *Systema Naturae* (1735*a*) and of the *Genera Plantarum* (1735*b*) was the most famous of the latter. Sydenham had already proposed a botanical model for his concept of disease and, moreover, botany and medicine were at the time closely connected.

Linné's classification of plants was based on two principles. In Nature there exist species, each constituting a finite, stable category, without continuity with the others; the discovery of the true categories can only be achieved by choosing the right criteria. Although Linné tried to apply his method to medicine in his *Genera Morborum* (1763), it was left to two doctors to propose the first 'natural' nosologies in which psychiatry had a significant part: one of them, Boissier de Sauvages, was living in Montpellier where he became Professor of botany at the medical school in 1752; the other, William Cullen, born in Glasgow, taught successively chemistry, physiology, and medicine in Edinburgh from 1755 onwards.

The *Nosologia Methodica* of Boissier de Sauvages (1768) and the *First Lines in the Practice of Physics* (1777–84) of Cullen had a common purpose – to establish a natural classification of diseases – but differed markedly in other respects. Boissier de Sauvages who claimed in the subtitle of his book that it was "based on the principles of Sydenham and the system of the botanists" adhered strictly to Linné's scheme. He described more than 2400 species which are named according to Linné's binary system and affirmed that "a disease consists of a cluster of several independent symptoms, named syndrome by the Greeks". In fact, his nosography is mostly a compilation of the works of his predecessors cast artificially in the Linnéan mould. The picturesque names of the 14 species included in the gender melancholia – *melancholia vulgaris, amatoria, religiosa, anglica, enthusiastica*, and so on – throw doubts about their allegedly 'natural' syndromic nature.

Although the work of Cullen has the same aim as the *Nosologia Methodica*, the classification of the Scottish author reflects a different tradition. The concept of 'nervous disease' had been introduced by Willis (1682) and by Sydenham (1682) to replace the old humoral theory. The predecessor of Cullen in Edinburgh, Robert Whytt, had brought together under the heading of nervous disease, hysteria, hypochondriasis, and the proteiform group of the 'simple nervous disorders' (Whytt, 1765). Cullen, following the same approach, takes aetiopathogenic mechanisms as the main criterion (Cullen, 1775). He opposes the 'local diseases' produced by a known and limited lesion, to the 'general diseases'. Among the latter he describes neuroses (a term he had already introduced in 1769) as due to a general involvement of the nervous system, affecting its functions. They are subdivided according to the function concerned and the way it is affected in comas, adynamies, spasms, and vesanies, the last one including mainly the different forms of insanity. The choice of the aetiopathogenic processes as the 'natural' criteria of classification and the introduction of the concept of neurosis remain the lasting contributions of Cullen to the domain of psychiatric nosology.

The clinical approach

It remains an undeniable fact that the founder of psychiatry as a medical discipline is Philippe Pinel, even if his role in the liberation of the insane from their chains has been rightly subjected in recent years to a critical reappraisal. The publication in 1801 of his *Medico-Philosophical Treatise on Mental Alienation or Mania* was hailed by the philosophers Maine de Biran and Hegel as a moment of great importance in the history of mankind; by making the study of madness a part of medicine, it had given to the insane the dignity of human beings. However, during his lifetime, Pinel was not merely considered as a psychiatric specialist, but was considered, in France, as the leading authority in general medicine. In 1798 he had published *Philosophical Nosography* in which he had proposed a classification of all known diseases, and this work, which went through many editions, remained a standard reference book for a whole generation of students.

A striking discrepancy exists between the *Philosophical Nosography* and the *Treatise on Mental Alienation*. The former is obviously inspired by Cullen, whose *First Lines in the Practice of Physics* had been translated by Pinel several years before. The same four classes of diseases are described; the fourth one, neuroses, being divided into the four sections proposed by Cullen.

In the *Treatise on Mental Alienation* the perspective is radically different. In the foreword, Pinel describes how he was compelled to divide the "alterations of the understanding" both to satisfy his "sense of order" and answer to the practical necessities of the management of the patients in the hospital. He considers now that the "arbitrary and incomplete classifications of Sauvages and Cullen", when put on trial, show their insufficiencies and he proposes his own, based on "a deep study of the symptoms" (Pinel, 1801, 1809). Mental alienation includes four species: melancholia, mania, dementia, and idiotism. This model deserves a close examination because it will have a lasting influence on the later systems. Three main points must be singled out.

Firstly, the limits of alienation are no longer the limits of the vesanies. What remains is what we would call today mental disorders of psychotic intensity. The reason for this is of a practical nature. Bicêtre and la Salpêtrière were asylums for the insane. They received only severely affected patients, whose behaviour was such that they required compulsory segregation; they were 'alienated' from society by their disease. They were the only patients who came under the observation and the care of the specialists who were, from then on, called alienists and later psychiatrists, and this situation lasted until the end of the 19th century. During that time psychiatric classifications were mostly concerned with psychoses.

The second point concerns the position of hysteria and hypochondriasis. For Cullen both were neuroses but did not belong to the subgroup of the vesanies. Pinel, who in his *Nosography* had maintained the general concept of neurosis, discarded the term in his *Treatise*. By excluding hysteria and hypochondriasis from his book he initiated a dichotomy in the field of mental disorders. Neurosis continued to be used to qualify a number of disturbances, but was completely dissociated from mental alienation. The new class of neurosis, deprived of the vesanies, was to have a complex history. It was defined by often changing criteria and lost progressively many of its original components which were attributed to the neurological, endocrinological, and even infectious diseases. Hysteria and hypochondriasis were the only survivors of Cullen's neuroses, but new entities were added such as neurasthenia, anxiety neurosis, phobic and obsessional neuroses, which corresponded to Whytt's 'simple nervous disorders' (Whytt, 1765). However, the important fact is that Pinel's *Treatise* left the study of neuroses to general medicine and, when it was born around 1850, to neurology. The most important contributions to the subject did not come from psychiatrists but from people such as Briquet, who was Professor of internal medicine, and Beard, Charcot, or Freud, who were neurologists, and the nosology of neuroses developed along largely independent lines.

A third peculiarity of Pinel's concepts is that they diverge fundamentally from those of Boissier de Sauvages and Cullen. Pinel did not accept Cullen's idea of the classifying role of an aetiopathogenic criterion. In the *Treatise* he abandons practically any coherent theory about the causes and mechanisms of insanity. In fact his main reference is the "deep study of the symptoms". Boissier de Sauvages had also claimed that his nosography was based essentially on symptoms. Pinel describes only four species and moreover does not really consider them as separate entities. They are but modes of expression of a single disease, mental alienation, as testified by the fact that in the title of his book, he uses the word in the singular (Pinel, 1801, 1809). His species do not have the ontological quality of Boissier de Sauvages' categories, they only provide a convenient instrument for the management of the patients. The idea of the unicity of insanity which in Pinel came from a pragmatic clinical and therapeutic attitude, and is in sharp contrast to the rigidly categorical scholastic approach of Boissier de Sauvages, was to reappear constantly later, on modified premises and in modified form.

In the words of Gourevitch (1983) "the mythical history of the birth of psychiatry in Paris makes a clinician the successor of a philanthropist. Pinel had delineated the limits of the field of psychiatry, Esquirol had transformed it in a garden of species". Pinel had in fact more preoccupations with nosology than his pupil Esquirol, even if he had largely abandoned them in his *Treatise*.

The greatness of Esquirol's work lies in the accuracy of his clinical descriptions far more than in his theoretical speculations. He recognised it when writing in the foreword of his textbook (1838): "I narrate the facts as I saw them. I have rarely sought to explain them and I have never tarried before systems which have always seemed to me to attract by their brilliance rather than be useful in their applications". He has followed Pinel's ideas in their broad outlines and, if his textbook is entitled *Treatise on the Mental Diseases*, it expresses more a concession to the medical habits than a deep conviction in the existence of finite categories of mental disorders. His main contribution to nosology concerns a specific domain: the revision of Pinel's melancholia. The state of the mood became the basic criterion and allowed to separate two species: lypemania whose primary manifestation was a 'pathological sadness'; and monomanias which regrouped the remaining cases. Lypemania could of course present delusional symptoms – Pinel had defined melancholia as a 'délire partiel' – but, if they existed, they were secondary to the abnormality of mood, and anyway their presence was not necessary. The new terminology did not survive but the conception of lypemania as a depression of mood was integrated in the post-Esquirolian melancholia.

The organic medical model

Both Pinel and Esquirol were extremely cautious when it came to incriminating lesions of the brain as causes of mental alienation. Pinel had little sympathy for Gall's doctrine and Esquirol was more interested in clinical observations than in the results of autopsies. It was left to a pupil of Esquirol, Georget, to introduce organicity as a principle of differentiation inside the global concept of insanity. In *On Madness* (1820) Georget admits the general postulate that any pathology of the mind implies the participation of the brain, but proposes to distinguish between two qualitatively different types of mental alienation. The first one, 'délire aigu' (acute delirium) whose manifestations express the cerebral reaction either to a direct toxic or cerebral involvement or indirectly to a somatic disease, is 'but a symptom'. The second one, 'madness', includes the species of mental alienation of Pinel and Esquirol, mania, melancholia, dementia and idiocy, to which he added a fifth one, the confusional curable state or 'stupidity'. It is easy to recognise in Georget's dichotomy the first draft of the later distinction between organic disorders and functional psychoses, even if his respect for the work of Esquirol compelled him to reluctantly maintain dementia and idiocy in the second group.

Two years after the publication of *On Madness*, in 1822, a young resident at the Charenton hospital near Paris, Bayle, presented and defended his inaugural thesis entitled *Research on Mental Diseases* (Bayle, 1822) in which he undertook to "prove that insanity is sometimes the symptom of chronic inflammation of the arachnoid". The description by Bayle of general paralysis is a landmark in the history of psychiatry. For the first time an entity was isolated and clinically characterised by specific symptoms having a definite course and aetiologically by a precise lesion of the central nervous system. The scheme corresponded perfectly with the concept of disease which, at the same time, was established in medicine by using the anatomo-clinical approach.

In 1826, in his *Treatise on Brain Diseases*, Bayle suggested that the model could also be applied to the understanding of madness, of the hitherto idiopathic alienation. The real turning-point came later, in 1855, with

Moreau de Tours who, taking general paralysis as an example, affirmed that one could describe 'mental entities' whose symptoms, whatever their nature – psychological or neurological – stemmed from the same lesion of the brain (Moreau de Tours, 1854–55). The scepticism of Pinel and Esquirol was now forgotten, and the neuropsychiatric perspective, whose emblem was general paralysis, took a leading position.

The search for a relation between symptoms and cause, illustrated by Bayle, was also, in a different perspective, the basis of the work of Morel. In Morel's epoch-making *Treatise on the Physical and Mental Degeneracies of the Human Species* (1857), he introduced the idea that a large part of mental alienation was but an expression of a functional and possibly lesional change of the nervous system produced by the process of degeneracy. Any psychological or physical noxious influence provokes, in the organism, a pathological deviation from the originally perfect state of humanity, and those deviations are inherited. Since the noxious influences are usually permanent, they have a cumulative effect and degenerative changes increase in severity with the successive generations of the affected family. Mental disorders, symptomatic of the common aetiological process, can be accordingly classified in a hierarchical way from the mildest, the 'nervous temperament', to the severest, 'idiocy'. Morel's conviction that nosology must only use causes as its criteria extended to the smaller part of mental pathology not accounted for by degeneracy.

In his *Treatise on Mental Diseases* (1860), Morel refused to consider melancholia and mania as "essential forms" since "depression and excitation are but symptoms which can be found in any form of madness". Morel's nosology has been important on several counts. It was the first comprehensive nosology claiming to be established on a purely aetiological basis. The concept of degeneracy, despite its scientific weakness due to the acceptance of the heredity of acquired characteristics, is, as Jaspers (1913) has pointed out, the origin of the later notion of endogeneity. Finally, Morel's mental diseases are no longer restricted to alienation. The mild manifestations of degeneracy include some of the symptoms of personality disorder and the classical neuroses are reintegrated in the psychiatric field.

Theories of classification

As the 19th century was nearing its end, psychiatric nosology entered its modern phase. The second edition of Kraepelin's textbook of psychiatry, published in 1887, and the sixth edition which appeared in 1899, present a striking contrast. One is still rooted in old concepts and uses an obsolete terminology, the other can be easily understood today.

Although the absence of real discontinuities in history makes division into periods largely arbitrary, one may reasonably consider that modern psychiatric nosologies were born about a century ago as the result of a long process during which empirical observations have been accumulated and theoretical interpretations proposed. It seems therefore fitting at this point, before describing the nosological models which are, in one form or another, still in existence, to discuss their logical aspects, their purposes, and their varieties.

Classification consists of dividing a population of elements into subpopulations according to certain rules which allow the attribution of each element to a definite category. Condensation of information is the basic purpose of the procedure. By knowing that an element belongs to a category, we know that it possesses a certain number of characteristics without enumerating them. Categories are defined by criteria which are chosen according to the purpose of the classification. A gardener will possibly classify plants according to their size, or the colour of their flowers, or any such property which will help in his/her work. Such classifications based on a single characteristic are said to be artificial. Although useful for special practical purposes, they allow only a limited prediction. A classification is said to be natural when its predictive value extends to the maximum possible number of facts and there is, for that reason, in any field of science, only one natural classification, based on the optimal combination of appropriate characteristics.

The criteria used for classification can belong to different levels, but if a classification based on superficial criteria is natural, it will hold true when, with the advances of knowledge, more basic theoretical criteria can be used. The original classification of plants based on their observable morphology was not substantially modified by the progresses of palaeontology and by the discovery of genes, nor was the Mendeleyev classification of elements, based on chemical reactivity, invalidated by the study of their atomic structure.

In psychiatry, as in medicine in general, criteria for classification pertain to three levels: those of the symptoms, of the mechanisms, and of the causes. This is, of course, an oversimplification; in psychiatry symptoms can be subjectively felt (symptoms *stricto sensu*) or be behavioural or somatic changes observed by the doctors (signs). It is also possible to take into account their temporal evolution; pathogenic criteria include both neurophysiological and biochemical brain processes and psychological mechanisms, and causes can belong to the psychological, social, or biological spheres. Nevertheless, one can schematically develop symptomatic, pathogenic, and aetiological nosologies, the last being viewed as hierarchically superior and considered as the really 'natural' ones.

Symptomatic categories are ideally syndromes. If in a population of individuals the frequency of symptom A is x, and the frequency of symptom B is y, a syndrome exists if the observed frequency of the subjects presenting simultaneously the two symptoms is significantly superior to the frequency x by y, which would be expected if the two symptoms were independent, the same reasoning being applicable to any cluster of symptoms. The relationships between the three levels are complex. A syndrome, as it has been defined, that is if it is not an arbitrary combination of symptoms, is the expression of a mechanism; but this mechanism may be triggered by one or several causes. Two additional remarks have to be made.

Firstly, most models are not homogeneous. They may combine elements from two or even three levels. This lack of homogeneity can express itself in another way. The field of psychiatry is divided into two or more fields, each submitted to a different nosological system: since Georget, the so-called organic disorders have been classified according to the known biological causes (or to a combination of symptoms and causes) whereas, in the remaining field, different, that is syndromic criteria, have been used.

The second remark concerns a general phenomenon in scientific classifications. The number of categories chosen depends to some extent on the personal inclination of the author whose attitude of mind orientates him/her towards a more analytic or more synthetic pole, as it is illustrated by the nosology of Boissier de Sauvages and that of Pinel.

Until now I have dealt with models derived from Sydenham's disease concept, which rests on the assumption that one can summarise the available information by describing finite classes of individuals, each being defined by a set of common characteristics. Since the early days of psychiatry, the legitimacy of such a categorical approach has been more or less openly questioned. Non-categorical views have not only been expressed in the traditional ambiguous formula – "There are no diseases, but only patients" – but they have been supported by philosophical theories and formalised in various models. The most extreme position rests on the work of Wilhelm Dilthey (1921–58) who opposed the natural sciences, whose function was to explain (*erklären*) observed events by relating them to other events in accordance with natural laws, and the sciences of the mind (*Geisteswissenschaften*), which are based on the direct understanding (*verstehen*) of the individual personality in its structure and history, each man being a law unto himself. As a consequence, psychology and, by extension, psychiatry must be idiographic and not nomothetic, that is, it must aim at the description of each individual and not at the discovery of general laws, which is implicitly the justification for the categorical approach.

Such a negative position, although with a different background and different implications, is apparent in dimensional models. The old psychological concept of the faculties of the soul had allowed the description of the expected behaviour of an individual by enumerating the strengths and weaknesses of each one. Laplace (1878–1912), Gauss (1821) and their successors made a mathematical formulation possible. The 'normal law' was shown by Quételet (1831) to fit the distribution of physical characteristics in the general population, and Francis Galton (1883) extended this observation to psychological features. The use of such a dimensional model has two consequences: being a continuous distribution, the difference between normality and pathology is not qualitative, but only quantitative; and there is a necessity to discover the most appropriate dimensions.

It was left to the British statisticians of the beginning of this century to propose an appropriate statistical technique by developing factor analysis. However, the dimensional approach had existed long before, and one can already consider Morel's degeneracy as a dimensional entity whose degrees of intensity are expressed in various pathological conditions. Between the idiographic and the dimensional approaches, many other intermediate non-categorical models have been proposed. One, which is still influential, stems from the work of Guislain who, in his *Treatise on Phrenopathies* (1835), suggested that all aspects of mental alienation were but subsequent reactions to a common 'fundamental alteration' – 'moral pain'.

The idea, taken over by Zeller who added the notion that the symptomatic reactions appear in a given sequence in the patient and belong to a 'unitary psychosis' (*Einheitspsychose*), was adopted by Griesinger (1845), and since then it has been detectable under various guises (Vliegen, 1980). Whatever the nature of the non-categorical model, its validity extends sometimes only to a fraction of the mental disorders. The *Einheitspsychose* involved only our functional psychoses and Morel opposed the 'accidental mental disorders' to the manifestations of degeneracy.

The concept of disease

Kraepelin's work occupies a central position among the models which have been proposed for a century and are still competing with each other. In the fifth edition of his *Treatise* (1896) he announced that from then on he would adopt an exclusively clinical perspective, which he elaborated in the 'concept of disease' (*Krankheitsbegriff*) based on the following principles (Hoff, 1985). They are, in psychiatry, finite categories – the diseases. If we had at our disposal all the scientific facts, we could define the categories either by symptomatic, pathogenic, or aetiological criteria, but the three resulting nosologies would be identical, a perfect correspondence between the three levels being postulated. Accordingly, if we do not yet have a sufficient knowledge of the mechanisms and of the causes, the study of the symptoms, of their conditions of apparition, their nature, and their evolution will result in a 'natural' nosology.

The emphasis on evolution, which was taken from Falret through Kahlbaum, allowed Kraepelin to describe and oppose dementia praecox (our schizophrenia) and the manic–depressive insanity, but his main contentions were the strictly categorical nature of nosology and the unequivocal nature of the relation between symptoms and causes. As far as the latter were concerned, his position was far from dogmatic. He accepted the existence of both psychological and biological factors and recognised that their nature and role were still in many cases hypothetical or unknown. The influence of Kraepelin's nosology remains considerable, not so much through the formulation of the *Krankheitsbegriff*, but because the categories the concept allowed him to describe clinically have remained, whatever the intervening modifications in their nomenclature and content: the direct precursors of our present-day mental disorders.

Two categorical models are related to Kraepelin's nosology. The first model, which was anterior to it, was proposed by Wernicke (1900) and postulated, in contrast to Kraepelin's cautious aetiological formulations, that each category has a biological basis in the form of a limited anatomical structure or of a physiological mechanism in the brain. Kraepelin condemned it ironically as a beautiful monument built on shaky foundations and it was for a time relatively forgotten. However, it kept its vitality, was developed by Kleist (1934) and, more recently, by Leonhard (1972); a specific heredity being postulated for all categories which, in contradistinction to Kraepelin's simple scheme, are numerous. This lasting influence expresses itself in many ways today. Leonhard's classification has enthusiastic proponents in some countries; concepts such as those of the unipolar and bipolar disorders and of the autonomous cycloid or schizoaffective psychoses derive directly from it. More broadly it can be said that some orientations of present-day biological psychiatry are closely connected to it: the use of the new brain imagery techniques has given arguments in its favour as, for instance, in the description of subtypes of schizophrenia or in the delimitation of the obsessive–compulsive disorder; and again the hypothesis that different reactions to different drugs are valid classification criteria, as in the panic and generalised anxiety disorders, rests on Wernicke's basic idea.

The second model, related to Kraepelin's nosology, and posterior to it, was elaborated by Kurt Schneider (1987). Its importance lies not only in the introduction of the 'first-rank symptoms', one of the sources of the diagnostic criteria, but also in the originality and clarity of its underlying principles. Psychiatry is divided into two fields, corresponding respectively to the 'diseases' and to the 'abnormal variations' with no transition between them. The former field, submitted to the categorical system, includes the pathological manifestations whose cause is biological, and is subdivided provisorily into two sections: the organic psychoses whose biological aetiology is already shown; and the endogenous ones, essentially schizophrenia and manic–depressive psychosis, whose biological origin is expressly affirmed (the so-called 'somatogenic postulate'). As we do not know the exact aetiology of the latter yet, their classification has to stay provisionally on the syndromic level: hence the description of the first-rank symptoms. Contrary to the 'diseases', the abnormal variations merge insensibly into the normal personality, and are but quantitatively different from it. They include the psychopathic personalities (our personality disorders) and the reactions to experience (*Erlebnisreaktionen*). The term neurosis is never used and the corresponding manifestations are included here. The model of the variations is purely dimensional and the descriptions based exclusively on symptoms. Since there is a continuum with normality, Schneider proposes as criteria for the existence of pathology the presence of suffering in the individual or in society.

The models of Wernicke, Kraepelin and Schneider, the last one only in the domain of his 'diseases', are categorical and postulate, each in its own way, a strong correlation between the patterns of symptoms and the causes. They are still with us, consciously or not, even if their influence may apparently concern the categories described on the basis of their theories rather than the theoretical background itself. But as soon as they appeared, doubts were raised about their validity. Hoche, the main opponent to Kraepelin's *Krankheitsbegriff* did accept the legitimacy of a categorical approach, but insisted on the possibility that the same cluster of symptoms could have several aetiologies. His 'syndromic doctrine' (*Syndromenlehre*) (Hoche, 1912) was of course in its principles as old as psychiatry, but has to be seen as an expression of the resistance to the disease concept. To a certain extent, the same can be said of Bleuler's clinical description of schizophrenia (Bleuler, 1911). Although acknowledging the value of Kraepelin's clinical description of dementia praecox, he adopted a profoundly different perspective. By establishing the diagnosis on the 'basic symptoms' (*Grundsymptome*), and not on a common evolution, by speaking in the title of his book of the "group of schizophrenias", he transformed the Kraepelinian 'disease' into a syndrome.

The non-categorical models

Psychiatric thinking has always balanced between two opposite poles, between the natural sciences and Dilthey's sciences of the mind, between a nomothetic categorisation of a medical nature and idiographic positions. The hostility to categorical models has been formulated in extremely different terms. We may mention here the existential analysis whose role has always remained limited, and Adolf Meyer's concept of 'reaction types' whose influence, especially on the psychiatry of the USA, must not be underestimated (Meyer, 1948–52).

However, the main anticategorical currents have their origin in two widely different domains: psychoanalysis and statistical psychology. It may appear ironical that among the first psychiatric contributions of Freud (1906), one finds the delimitation of a new entity, the anxiety neurosis, defined by the traditional combination of a cluster of symptoms, a pathogeny, and an assumedly biological cause. However, Freud was not deeply interested in nosology and his main efforts concentrated on the psychological mechanisms which, in relation to maturation and early life situations, were responsible for the appearance of pathological symptoms. Psychoanalysis accepted more or less the established nosology without giving much thought to it. But its concentration on the level of psychological mechanisms, the evolution of the diverging schools of 'dynamic psychiatry', have led many of its adherents to reject any categorical model, as evidenced by the statement of Masserman (1953) who condemns "the tendency to 'define' and classify 'mental disorders' into categories comparable to those used in general medicine, despite the fact that in the case of most mental disorders, little justification for such a classification exists on aetiologic, clinical and even heuristic grounds".

A formalisation of the dimensional approach, another less extreme expression of the anticategorical attitude, was made possible by the introduction of factor analysis by Spearman in 1904. It was first applied to psychiatry by Moore (1929) but had been, for a long time, used by psychologists to discover the basic dimensions allowing a meaningful description of any individual's personality in a system of reference. After 1950 many attempts were made at a dimensional description of psychiatric symptoms, thanks to the parallel development of psychiatric rating scales and to the technical facilities offered by modern computers. The term syndrome, frequently attributed by American authors to such dimensions, is misleading, since syndromes in the medical sense can only be isolated by another multivariate mathematical procedure, cluster analysis. The most ambitious of the dimensional models, encompassing the whole of psychiatry, have been proposed by psychologists – Eysenck's tridimensional model being one of the best known (Eysenck, 1955). But the approach has also been intensively applied by psychiatrists to limited domains.

The controversy about the existence, either of distinct categories inside the anxiety and depressive disorders or of a continuum, which has opposed psychiatrists mainly in the UK, has made great use of arguments derived from such mathematical methods. The current discussions about the optimal number of dimensions to be used in the description of schizophrenic symptoms are another example.

The DSM–III approach

The success of the third edition of the *Diagnostic and Statistical Manual of Mental Disorders* (DSM–III; American Psychiatric Association, 1980) and adoption of its principles in ICD–10 (World Health Organization, 1992) may infer that we have reached the end of the history of the competing nosological models in psychiatry. Much has been and is still written about the DSM–III and only some important points will be evoked. Although the authors state that "there is no assumption that each mental disorder is a discrete entity", the categorical nature of the system is the natural result of the use of diagnostic criteria, introduced for improving the interrater reliability of the diagnoses. This categorical nature is the only justification for the qualification of 'neo-Kraepelinian', much used in the USA by some of the authors of DSM–III. The extension of a categorical model to the whole field of mental pathology is the source of difficulties.

Personality disorders are expressedly described as exaggerations of personality traits, but the logical consequence, drawn by Kurt Schneider of the adoption of a dimensional model (Schneider, 1987), has been eluded since "traditionally the clinician has been directed to find a single personality disorder that adequately describes the person's disturbed personality functioning", the result being that a single diagnosis is frequently completed with difficulty.

The main claim of the DSM–III is its 'atheoretical' nature. Except for the organic disorders and a few psychogenic reactions, the categories are described by symptomatic criteria; no hypothesis being made, at least theoretically, about the generally 'unproved' aetiopathogeny. It is a direct repudiation of Wernicke, Kraepelin and Schneider, together with some psychoanalytic conceptions. In its selection of syndromal categories, the DSM–III has made some innovations which, in conjunction with the adoption of a few new terms, has been a source of discussion, but they have not been of a fundamental nature. A conspicuous trend has been the increase in their number, accentuated in the revised edition (DSM–III–R; American Psychiatric Association, 1987).

This analytic position, whose justification is the necessity of increasing the homogeneity of the pathological groups, leaves open two basic questions: are the criteria selected significant ones; and do the clusters of symptoms chosen correspond to the statistical definition of a syndrome? The answer depends on the 'natural' or 'artificial' nature of the classification proposed. The wide acceptance of the DSM–III and of the related ICD–10 is largely due to the fact that they provide a practical answer to the need for a common language in psychiatry. But the application of such a detailed categorical classification of high reliability to such crucial domains as epidemiology and clinical psychopharmacology, for which it was presented as especially appropriate, has already raised doubts about its validity. The incidence of comorbidity between categories in many epidemiological studies reaches a level which has no equivalent in other branches of medicine and suggests the need for a reappraisal of the categorical structure. The relative lack of a precise and direct correspondence between nosological categories and the efficacy of chemically and pharmacologically specific drugs have led to the suggestion that a better understanding could proceed from a trans-nosological approach. Such criticisms are not of a theoretical nature, but rest on the objective results of concrete applications.

Conclusions

The numerous problems raised by the multiplicity of nosological approaches can be reduced to a few basic questions. Does psychiatry constitute a homogeneous field which has to be submitted to the same model? If the answer is no, which model is the most appropriate to each subgroup of mental disorders? Nosologies, in every branch of medicine, are attempts of the integration of the available knowledge in a construct which, to varying degrees, implies hypotheses. The present trend claims to favour the former and to condemn the latter. However, it must not be forgotten that the value of a nosology is gauged by the number of predictions it allows, and that nosological concepts based on speculative views have often proved to be useful.

A perfect psychiatric nosology is probably an unattainable goal, but a better consciousness of the nature of the models which have been successively proposed and are still largely with us could help our progress in its direction.

References

AMERICAN PSYCHIATRIC ASSOCIATION (1980) *Diagnostic and Statistical Manual of Mental Disorders* (3rd edn) (DSM-III). Washington, DC: APA.
—— (1987) *Diagnostic and Statistical Manual of Mental Disorders* (3rd edn, revised) (DSM-III-R). Washington, DC: APA.
BAYLE, A. L. J. (1822) Recherches sur les maladies mentales (thèse de Médecine, Paris). In *Centenaire de la Thèse de Bayle*. Paris: Masson (1922).
—— (1826) *Traité des Maladies du Cerveau et de ses Membranes*. Paris: Gabon.
BLEULER, E. (1911) *Dementia Praecox oder Gruppe der Schizophrenien*. Leipzig/Wien: F. Deuticke.
BOISSIER DE SAUVAGES, F. (1768) *Nosologia Methodica, Sistens Morborum Classes, Genera et Species Juxta Sydenhami Mentem et Botanicorum Ordinem*. Amsterdam: de Tournes.
CULLEN, W. (1775) *Apparatus ad Nosologiam Methodicam seu Synopsis Nosologicae Methodicae in Usum Studiorum*. Amsterdam: de Tournes (1st edn, Edinburgh, 1769).
—— (1777-84) *First Lines in the Practice of Physics*. Edinburgh: Elliott.
DILTHEY, W. (1921-58) *Gesammelte Schriften*. Leipzig: Teubner.
ESQUIROL, E. (1838) *Des Maladies Mentales Considérées sous les Rapports Médical, Hygiénique et Médico-Légal*. Paris: Baillière.
EYSENCK, H. J. (1955) Psychiatric diagnosis as a psychological and statistical problem. *Psychological Reports*, **1**, 3-17.
FREUD, S. (1906) *Sammlung kleiner Schriften zur Neurosenlehre aus den Jahren 1894-1906*. Leipzig/Wien: Franz Deuticke.
GALTON, F. (1883) *Inquiry into Human Faculty and its Development*. London: Cassell.
GAUSS, C. F. (1821) Theoria combinationis observationum erroribus minimis obnoxiae. Pars prior. In *Carl Friedrich Gauss Werke* (1980), pp. 1-26, 85-1000. Göttingen: Dietrische Universitätsdruckerei.
GEORGET, E. (1820) *De la Folie*. Paris: Crevot.
GOUREVITCH, M. (1983) Esquirol et la nosologie. In *Nouvelle Histoire de la Psychiatrie* (eds J. Postel & C. Quétel). Toulouse: Privat.

GRIESINGER, W. (1845) *Die Pathologie und Therapie der Psychischen Krankheiten für Aerzte und Studierende.* Stuttgart: Adolph Krabbe.

GUISLAIN, J. (1835) *Traité des Phrénopathies ou Doctrine Nouvelle des Maladies Mentales* (2nd edn). Bruxelles: Etablissement encyclographique.

HOCHE, A. H. (1912) Die Bedeutung der Symptomenkomplexe in der Psychiatrie. *Zeitschrift für die Gesamte Neurologie und Psychiatrie,* **12,** 540–551.

HOFF, P. (1985) Zum Kranheitsbegriff bei Emil Kraepelin. *Nervenarzt,* **56,** 510–513.

JASPERS, K. (1913) *Allegemeine Psychopathologie.* Berlin: Springer.

KLEIST, K. (1934) *Gehirnpathologie.* Leipzig: J. A. Barth.

KRAEPELIN, E. (1887) *Psychiatrie. Ein kurzes Lehrbuch für Studirende und Aerzte* (2nd edn). Leipzig: Ambr. Abel.

—— (1896) *Psychiatrie. Ein Lehrbuch für Studirende und Aerzte* (5th edn). Leipzig: J. A. Barth.

—— (1899) *Psychiatrie. Ein Lehrbuch für Studirende und Aerzte* (6th edn). Leipzig: J. A. Barth.

LAPLACE, P. S. DE (1878–1912) *Oeuvres Complètes.* Paris: Gauthier-Villars.

LEONHARD, K. (1972) Aufteilung der endogenen Psychosen in der Forschungsrichtung von Wernicke und Kleist. In *Psychiatrie der Gegenwart. Forschung und Praxis. Band II. Teil l. Klinische Psychiatrie* (2nd edn) (eds K. P. Kisker, J. E. Meyer, M. Müller & E. Strömgren). Berlin: Springer.

LINNÉ, C. VON (1735a) *Systema Naturae Sive Regna tri a Naturae Systematica Proposita per Clases, Ordines, Genera et Species.* Leyden: J. Haak.

—— (1735b) *Genera Plantarum Eaorumque Characteres Naturales, Secundum Numerum, Figurem, Sitium et Proportionem Omnium Fructificationis Partum.* Leyden: C. Wishoff.

—— (1763) *Genera Morborum in Auditorum Usum.* Uppsala: C. E Steinart.

MASSERMAN, J. E. (1953) *Principles of Dynamic Psychiatry.* Philadelphia: W. B. Saunders.

MEYER, A. (1948–52) *Collected Papers of Adolf Meyer.* Baltimore: Johns Hopkins University Press.

MOORE, T. V. (1929) The empirical determination of certain syndromes underlying praecox and manic–depressive psychoses. *American Journal of Psychiatry,* **9,** 719–738.

MOREAU DE TOURS, J. (1854–55) Du délire au point de vue pathologique et anatomo-pathologique. *Bulletin de l'Académie Impériale de Médecine,* **20,** 908–917.

MOREL, B. A. (1857) *Traité des Dégénérescences Physiques, Intellectuelles et Morales de l'Espèce Humaine et des Causes qui Produisent ces Varieétes Maladives.* Paris: Baillière.

—— (1860) *Traité des Maladies Mentales.* Paris: Masson.

PINEL, P. (1798) *Nosographie Philosophique ou la Méthode de l'Analyse Appliquée à la Médecine.* Paris: Maradon.

—— (1801) *Traité Médico-Philosophique sur l'Aliénation Mentale ou la Manie.* Paris: Richard, Caille et Ravier.

—— (1809) *Traité Médico-Philosophique sur l'Aliénation Mentale.* Paris: Brosson.

QUÉTELET, A. (1831) *Recherches sur la Loi de la Croissance de l'Homme.* Bruxelles: Haez.

SCHNEIDER, K. (1987) *Klinische Psychopathologie* (12th edn). Stuttgart: G. Thieme.

SPEARMAN, C. E. (1904) "General intelligence" objectively determined and measured. *American Journal of Psychology,* **15,** 201–293.

SYDENHAM, T. (1682) *Dissertatio Epistolaris ad C. Cole de observationis Nuperis Circa Curationem Variolarum Confluentium, Necnam de Affectione Hysterica.* London: Kettelby.

VLIEGEN, J. (1980) *Die Einheitspsychose. Geschichte und Probleme.* Stuttgart: F. Enke.

WERNICKE, C. (1900) *Grundriss der Psychiatrie.* Leipzig: G. Thieme.

WHYTT, R. (1765) *Observations on the Nature, Causes and Cure of those Disorders which are Commonly Called Nervous, Hypochondriac and Hysteric.* Edinburgh: Becket and De Hondt.

WILLIS, T. (1682) *Opera Omnia.* Amsterdam: Wetstenius.

WORLD HEALTH ORGANIZATION (1992) *The ICD–10 Classification of Mental and Behavioural Disorders.* Geneva: WHO.

2 Myself and my other self: the "double phenomenon" in neurotic disorders

ANDREW SIMS

"He had two selves within him apparently, and they must learn to accommodate each other and their reciprocal impediments. Strange, that some of us, with quick alternate vision, see beyond our infatuations, and even while we rave on the heights, behold the wide plain where our persistent self pauses and awaits us". George Eliot, 1871, *Middlemarch*.

The 'double'

There has been considerable confusion in psychiatric writing between (a) heautoscopy, autoscopy, and phantom mirror image (these are synonyms); (b) the 'double' phenomenon, which is the subject of this chapter; and (c) dual, double, or multiple personality. There is not usually confusion in distinguishing psychopathologically between the 'double' phenomenon and others such as delusional misidentification, the Capgras' syndrome and its variants, and double orientation.

Jaspers (1959) stated:

"Heautoscopy is the term used for the phenomenon when someone vividly perceives his own body as a double in the outer world, whether as an actual perception or as an imaginary form, as a delusion or as a vivid physical awareness. There have been patients who will actually speak with their doubles. The phenomenon is not at all uniform."

He gives, for example, four cases of patients, one of whom is suffering from an organic condition, two from schizophrenia, and one definitely not organic, and then goes on to write:

"We can see that we are dealing with phenomena that are really not the same although they are superficially similar. They may occur in organic brain lesions, in deliria, in schizophrenia and in dream-like states, never at least without

18

a mild alteration in consciousness; day-dreaming, intoxication, dream-sleep or delirium. The similarity consists in the fact that the body-schema gains an actuality of its own out in external space.''

It would seem that Jaspers is here describing two separate phenomena: autoscopy and the 'double' phenomenon. Autoscopy or phantom mirror image has been described by Fish (1967):

> ''In this strange experience the patient sees himself and knows that it is he. It is not just a visual hallucination because kinaesthetic and somatic sensations must also be present to give the subject the impression that the hallucination is he.''

Alternatively, Lukianowicz (1958) stated:

> ''Autoscopy is a complex psychosensorial hallucinatory perception of one's own body image projected into the external visual space.''

These descriptions of autoscopy imply that the experience is perceptual, involving loss of the feeling of familiarity for one's self. Visual hallucinations are invariable, and there may be other features. The condition is often associated with parietal lobe lesion.

By contrast, Jaspers' first example of the 'double' came from Goethe – to quote Jaspers quoting Goethe:

> ''Goethe (in *Drang und Verwirrung*) had seen Frederika for the last time and was riding to Drusenheim when the following happened: 'In my mind's eye, not with my physical eyes, I saw myself distinctly on the same road riding towards myself. I was dressed as I had never been before in grey and gold. Immediately I shook myself out of this dream the figure went' . . . 'the strange phantom gave me a certain peace of mind at that moment of parting'. What is noteworthy in the episode is the dreamy state, the mind's eye and the satisfaction derived from the meaning of the apparition – he was riding in the opposite direction back to Sesenheim – he will return.''

Despite Menninger-Lerchenthal's (1932) title of the relevant paper *An Hallucination of Goethe*, this was certainly not an hallucination; it is described as ''in my mind's eye''. It is not organic, neither is it psychotic; it is, in fact, a description of fantasy. It would seem that there could be six possible psychopathological explanations for this phenomenon of non-organic, non-psychotic doubling:

(a) *Fantasy*, as in this description by Goethe of day-dreaming;
(b) *Depersonalisation*: . . . ''while talking we may notice that we are talking rather like an automaton, quite correctly maybe, but we can observe ourselves and listen to ourselves'' (Jaspers, 1959);

(c) *Conflict*: "Two beings live within my breast where reason struggles with passion" (Jaspers, 1959);

(d) *Compulsive ideas*: repetitive, self-produced and self-ascribed, resisted;

(e) *Double personality*, with alternating states of consciousness;

(f) *Being doubled*: "When both chains of psychic events so develop together that we can talk of separate personalities, each with their own peculiar experiences and specific feeling–associations, and each perfectly alien and apart from the other" (Jaspers, 1959).

These experiences are not wholly distinct from each other, and they do overlap; however, there are phenomenological differences between them that are important.

Multiple personality

Recently there has been a vast outpouring in the psychiatric literature on the subject of multiple personality disorder (MPD). Unfortunately, not all of this has been of high quality, and it has added to the confusion surrounding terminology. The diagnostic criteria of DSM–III–R (American Psychiatric Association, 1987) often appear to have been used without precision and without application of phenomenological principles. MPD has often been assumed to be a dissociative phenomenon.

This literature has been well summarised by Fahy (1988):

"Recently there has been a dramatic rise in the number of case reports of multiple personality disorder (MPD). . . . a review of the recent literature reveals a poverty of information on reliability of diagnosis, problems, or the role of selection bias. It is argued that iatrogenic factors may contribute to the development of the syndrome. There is little evidence from genetic or physiological studies to suggest that MPD represents a distinct psychiatric disorder."

The literature on multiple personality disorder, when reviewed phenomenologically, varies from quite clear dissociative phenomena to descriptions of the experience of being doubled. Slater & Roth (1969) succinctly commented:

"A girl who is by turns 'May' and 'Margaret', may be quiet, studious and obedient as May, and unaware of Margaret's existence. When she becomes Margaret, however, she may be gay, headstrong and wilful and refer to May in contemptuous terms. It seems that these multiple personalities are always artificial productions, the product of the medical attention that they arouse."

Phenomenology

In *General Psychopathology*, Jaspers (1959) defined phenomenology 30 or 40 times but always with the implication that it is the study of the *subjective* state by the use of *empathy*.

"Phenomenology involves the observation and categorisation of abnormal psychic events, the internal experiences of the patient and his consequent behaviour. An attempt is made to observe and understand the psychic event or phenomenon, so that the observer can, as far as possible, know for himself what the patient's experience must feel like" (Sims, 1988).

In his descriptions of the characteristics of *abnormal self-awareness*, Jaspers differentiates between the different abnormalities and describes 'disorder of the unity of self':

"Normally I am aware of myself as a unity. Psychopathologically I may be aware of myself as split up in some way, as no longer a unitary self. This is the real experience of being in two" (Walker, 1992).

This neurotic thinking, in Jaspers' terminology, is both 'reflective' and 'mediated', whereas schizophrenic 'made thoughts' are 'immediate' and 'immediated'. This double phenomenon is not dissociative, in that each part of the self is opposed to but aware of the other.

Examples of 'the double'

Figure 2.1 shows a simplified representation of the repertory grid provided by a 22-year-old female student, who introspected: "I can't cope . . . I get worked up about little things, anxious and guilty about leaving my parents and coming to university . . . everything is weighing me down". She described a very bad relationship between her parents who used to "play her off against each other". She was also perfectionistic.

"It was my problem, I thought I could work it out myself. I put on a false face with friends . . . that's not the real me. When I'm with people I'm talking and laughing with them, I don't feel comfortable. There is something inside myself watching myself, listening to myself . . . it is saying this is not me, this is not me. Perhaps it is the real me. The one inside is the real me. It is critical and says about the one being childish, why are you acting like this?".

This two-dimensional form of the repertory grid represents the subjective, semantic space of the patient by relating *elements* and *constructs*, which come from words and phrases that the patient has actually used. Elements are nouns, and in these cases, were significant people in the patient's

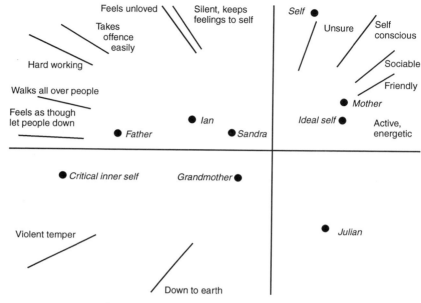

Fig. 2.1. Simplified repertory grid for a female student

environment, including different concepts of 'self'. Constructs are the adjectival descriptions of these elements. Elements are represented by points in space, and constructs by lines. The axes are mathematical abstractions; it is the relationships between elements and constructs that are important, and in these cases, especially the different descriptions of self.

Another patient, a successful barrister, described long-term difficulties with his relationships dating back to the death of his father when he was a child, and an over-close relationship subsequently with mother, sister and wife. He described experiencing himself as two quite different people, characterised as "the successful, international figure" and "the little boy who can't make up his mind". The *elements* (the significant people in his environment) and the *construct* (the way he regarded these people) are represented in the repertory grid of Fig. 2.2.

A third patient was reminiscent of *Death of a Salesman* by Arther Miller (1949). This was a 45-year-old male patient, previously highly successful as a salesman. Two years before admission he had left his job, his home, his wife and two children and drifted around the country, being admitted for short periods of time to several psychiatric hospitals. He described his subjective state:

"I feel very anxious, uncomfortable and depressed. It is like having the same person in the same body as me. It is like two different people inside one body.

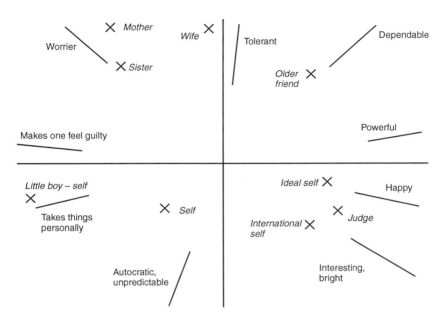

Fig. 2.2. Simplified repertory grid for a successful male barrister

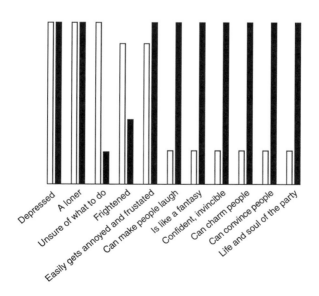

Fig. 2.3. 'Myself and my other self' – the two personalities of a previously successful salesman (□ myself, ■ other self)

One person is holding back – that's like me. The other person is trying to let go – the other is different, quite strong".

"Me" was described as "frightened, depressed, unsure", and "other" as "confident, affable, a great salesman". 'Self' and his 'other self' are compared in Fig. 2.3.

Comment

Clear descriptions of the non-psychotic 'double' are found in classical literature, such as Dostoievsky's *The Double* (1846) and *The Brothers Karamazov* (1879–80) where the brothers are different aspects of the self polarised. R. L. Stevenson has also portrayed this in *The Strange Case of Doctor Jekyll and Mr Hyde* (1886), as the best known example, but perhaps more interestingly in *The Master of Ballantrae* (1889), where once again the two brothers appear to be polarised representations of the same self:

> "'He will not show his face here again', said I. 'Oh yes he will', said Mr Henry. 'Where I am, there will he be'''.

The very worst feature of 'the double' for the subject himself is the terrible, inextricable involvement of the double with the subject in trying to mortify him, goad him, and provoke him to destroy the double and/or destroy himself. This destructiveness in severe depressive illness was described by Styron (1991):

> ". . . the sense of being accompanied by a second self – a wraith-like observer, able to watch with dispassionate curiosity as his companion struggles against the oncoming disaster, or decides to embrace it . . . I, the victim-to-be of self-murder, was both the solitary actor and lone member of the audience . . . I watched myself in mingled terror and fascination . . ."

Treatment

Even in such a brief survey, a number of useful principles can be established. The 'self' should be explored to ascertain the relationships of different selves. For this the phenomenological, empathic method is appropriate. Any other treatable psychiatric condition should be assessed: for example, depressive illness requires specific treatment.

The patient should be helped to accept, using a cognitive approach, that both selves are himself – and both essentially are parts of self. He should be helped to integrate the selves and draw them closer to 'self' and 'ideal self'. The repertory grid may be useful in making this approximation graphic and literal.

Conclusions

The double experience is phenomenologically distinct from autoscopy and multiple personality disorder (MPD). It occurs as a part of the disturbance of self-awareness, as a disorder of unity, in the phenomenology of neurotic disorders. 'Selves' are alien to, but may be aware of, each other.

Treatment may be beneficial, both directed at the disorder of self and any other psychiatric condition present.

References

AMERICAN PSYCHIATRIC ASSOCIATION (1987) *Diagnostic and Statistical Manual of Mental Disorders* (3rd edn, revised) (DSM–III–R). Washington, DC: APA.

DOSTOIEVSKY, F. M. (1846) *The Double* (trans. C. Garnett, 1913). St Petersburg: *The Literary Journal*.

—— (1879–80) *The Brothers Karamazov* (trans. C. Garnett, 1912). London: Heinemann.

ELIOT, G. (1871) *Middlemarch*. Edinburgh: William Blackwood.

FAHY, T. A. (1988) The diagnosis of multiple personality disorder: a critical review. *British Journal of Psychiatry*, **153**, 597–606.

FISH, F. (1967) *Clinical Psychopathology*. Bristol: John Wright.

JASPERS, K. (1959) *General Psychopathology* (7th edn) (trans. J. Hoenig & M. W. Hamilton, 1963). Manchester: Manchester University Press.

LUKIANOWICZ, N. (1958) Autoscopic phenomena. *Archives of Neurology and Psychiatry*, **80**, 199–220.

MENNINGER-LERCHENTHAL, E. (1932) Eine Halluzination Goethes. *Zeitschrift für die Gesamte Neurologie und Psychiatrie*, **140**, 486–495.

MILLER, A. (1949) *Death of a Salesman*. London: Cresset.

SIMS, A. C. P. (1988) *Symptoms in the Mind: An Introduction to Descriptive Psychopathology*. London: Baillière Tindall.

SLATER, E. & ROTH, M. (1969) *Clinical Psychiatry: Mayer Gross, Slater & Roth* (3rd edn). London: Baillière, Tindall & Cassell.

STEVENSON, R. L. (1886) *The Strange Case of Dr Jekyll and Mr Hyde*. London: Longman Green.

—— (1889) *The Master of Ballantrae*. London: Cassel.

STYRON, W. (1991) *Darkness Visible*. London: Jonathan Cape.

3 Defining the phenotype for molecular genetic research

ANNE E. FARMER and JULIE WILLIAMS

One of the current major concerns in biological psychiatry is the attempt to discover the molecular basis of schizophrenia, manic–depressive disorder and the other 'functional' psychoses. The impetus has been provided by 'classic' genetic studies using family, twin and adoption methods, which have demonstrated a genetic contribution to schizophrenia (Gottesman, 1991) and a variety of other disorders (McGuffin & Murray, 1991). The most common molecular genetic strategy is to take a positional cloning approach, in which genes are first located by linkage studies that investigate the cosegregation of genetic markers and the disorder in multiply-affected families. This is followed by a variety of techniques to focus in on the genes themselves and discover their structure, DNA sequence and their positive products. Positional cloning has been dramatically successful in single gene disorders, but has so far not progressed beyond the source for linkage in psychiatric disorders. This is probably because the mode of inheritance of a disorder like schizophrenia is complex and there is likely to be genetic heterogeneity, so that large sample sizes will probably be required to detect the relevant genes.

Large samples of multiply-affected families are best obtained by multi-centre collaboration, and recently large scale programmes have been set up in Europe under the auspices of the European Science Foundation (ESF) and in the US by the National Institutes of Health (NIH) (Leboyer & McGuffin, 1991). Such collaborations have implications for laboratory and clinical field work, in that both must be carried out in an economical and reliable way which ensures comparability of all data in all centres. Here we will focus on the methods used in the collection of clinical data. This has implications beyond genetics to other biological and epidemiological studies, and we will therefore begin by reviewing some of the more general issues in standardised approaches to psychiatric classification and diagnosis.

Establishing psychiatric diagnosis

Defining psychiatric disorder operationally is now virtually mandatory for research studies where the authors wish to publish their results in reputable journals. Since their introduction in the 1970's, operational definitions of psychiatric disorder have enhanced the reliability of diagnosis (Farmer *et al*, 1987). This has been largely brought about by their highly prescriptive 'top down' formats; that is, a series of pre-set fixed rules (criteria) have to be fulfilled before the diagnostic category can be applied. Agreement between raters regarding whether a subject fulfils the rules or not has been shown to be good (McGuffin *et al*, 1991). However, individuals who fail to fulfil one or more items fall outside the diagnosis and often end up in 'not elsewhere specified' or 'atypical' categories. If the criteria are too narrow, the majority of subjects end up in such categories, which may be larger than the main diagnostic groups (Farmer *et al*, 1992).

Another difficulty with operational definitions of psychiatric disorder is that the items included are rather limited and often focus on the more easily rated aspects of disorder. For example, definitions of schizophrenia seldom include negative features of the illness, such as amotivation and inappropriate or restricted affect, and concentrate on more readily rateable items such as delusions and hallucinations. The presence of a positive family history for the disorder and previous response to medication may also influence the diagnosis clinically, but are very seldom included in operational definitions.

The first set of operational definitions published were the St Louis criteria (Feighner *et al*, 1972). These were soon followed by the Research Diagnostic Criteria (Spitzer *et al*, 1975), the *Diagnostic and Statistical Manual of Mental Disorders* revised (DSM–III–R; American Psychiatric Association, 1987) and most recently by the Diagnostic Criteria for Research of the 10th edition of the *International Classification of Diseases* (ICD–10; World Health Organization, 1992). Because of their explicit format, it is possible to devise structured interviews, also 'top down' in design, to elicit the component items. Interviews based on the above definitions include the Schedule of Affective Disorders and Schizophrenia (SADS-LA; Mannuzza *et al*, 1986), and the Composite International Diagnostic Interview (CIDI; Robins *et al*, 1988).

Other types of interview also include operationally defined disorders within their coding algorithms. The Schedule for the Clinical Assessment of Neuropsychiatry (SCAN) is a more flexible style of interview which, although arriving at DSM–III–R and ICD–10 operational definitions, is not restricted by these diagnostic schema (Wing *et al*, 1990). SCAN incorporates a more 'bottom-up' approach, which starts with individual symptoms and attempts to find a diagnosis that will accommodate them. In practice, both styles of interview have been employed in molecular genetics research, with good agreement being found between them. For example, both SCAN and

SADS-LA are accepted as part of the minimum data set by the ESF Programme. They have also been shown to have reasonable levels of agreement in relation to psychotic disorders, with raters from different ESF collaborating countries (Farmer *et al*, 1993).

However, while the advantage of using operational criteria is improved interrater diagnostic reliability, enthusiasm for this approach must be tempered by disappointing agreement between different sets of criteria. Brockington *et al* (1978) and Stephens *et al* (1982) both found the diagnosis of schizophrenia to show differences between different operational criteria. This position was encapsulated by Brockington *et al*, who commented that the previous state of inarticulate confusion in the diagnosis of schizophrenia had been replaced by a ''babble of precise but differing formulations of the same concept''. In the face of such problems, Kendell (1975) suggested that a polydiagnostic approach be adopted in biological research. In practical terms this would mean that researchers would select one set of operational criteria, such as DSM–IV (American Psychiatric Association, 1994), to act as their main 'working hypothesis', but would collect sufficient information to fulfil the requirements of the other sets of operational criteria. This approach offers two initial advantages. The first is the opportunity for enhanced comparability between pieces of research which may have used different 'main' criteria, and the second is that it allows the differential utility of each set of criteria to be compared. To facilitate such a polydiagnostic approach, the Operational Criteria (OPCRIT) checklist and a suite of associated computer programs were devised (McGuffin *et al*, 1991).

The OPCRIT system

The OPCRIT checklist comprises 90 items of psychopathology, premorbid and personal data, and family history information. Together this information forms the basis for a diagnosis of a major psychiatric disorder under each of several classificatory systems (Feighner *et al*, 1972; Spitzer *et al*, 1975; Taylor & Abrams, 1978; American Psychiatric Association, 1987, 1994; World Health Organization, 1992), two commonly applied definitions of psychotic disorder (Schneider, 1959; Carpenter *et al*, 1973), a version of the French criteria for non-affective psychosis (Pull *et al*, 1987) and three additional subtypings of schizophrenia (Tsuang & Winokur, 1974; Crow, 1980; Farmer *et al*, 1983). The checklist information is entered into the OPCRIT computer package, which provides a detailed definition for each of the checklist items (McGuffin *et al*, 1991) and produces a series of diagnoses according to algorithms based upon the original operational criteria. OPCRIT is designed to be used by a clinician, with information obtained from any diagnostic interview, case notes and any other information which is of relevance. OPCRIT interrater reliability shows better than chance agreement, whether one compares ratings of individual checklist items or the ultimate diagnoses for each system of classification, with kappa scores ranging between 0.4 and 1 for the former and 0.57 and 0.87 for the latter (McGuffin *et al*, 1991). OPCRIT has been adopted as part of the minimum data set by both the ESF and the collaboration in the US sponsored by the National Institute of Mental Health (NIMH). Subsequently a new version of OPCRIT (3.3) has been designed for these collaborations, and a reliability study was commissioned by the ESF to encompass raters from all the European centres involved in the collaboration.

Although much work has gone into solving some of the problems associated with psychiatric diagnosis for molecular genetic research, other difficulties remain. These fall into two general categories – those associated with the operational definitions and those with the requirements of molecular genetic research. It is to these problems and their possible solutions we now turn.

Diagnosis and genetic research

One of the most difficult problems in the use of operational criteria for linkage and association studies is the almost total lack of a coherent and detailed hierarchy governing the production of a single diagnosis from the many defined within the classification system. That is, it is possible for a subject to fulfil the criteria for two or more disorders simultaneously. As a result, much attention has been focused on the finding of 'comorbidity' in clinical and epidiomological studies. For the most part, however, genetic studies require a simple, clear-cut affected/unaffected dichotomy. This posed a particular difficulty for the development of the computer algorithms for OPCRIT, but was overcome by specifying that where the hierarchy was unclear in the original published criteria, the diagnostic hierarchy suggested by Foulds (1965) was used. In other research or clinical settings, adopting a comorbid approach to diagnosis may be more appropriate. This has also been incorporated into the polydiagnostic approach in the form of an extension to OPCRIT in a program called OPCOM.

The lack of detailed specifications of the hierarchical elements embedded in the operational criteria, such as the predominance of psychotic or affective symptomatology, has resulted in decisions which are overtly dependent on clinical judgement. This has caused increased variability between diagnoses which are reliant on this subjective type of decision (Farmer *et al*, 1992) and was well illustrated in a recent ESF sponsored workshop in Mainz, Germany, on diagnosis within the ESF collaboration. Following a video presentation of a structured interview with a patient who displayed both affective and psychotic symptoms, the audience of European psychiatrists were asked to rate the relationship between psychotic and affective symptoms. Just under half considered that the symptoms appeared in a balanced relationship (which would result in a schizoaffective diagnosis using most sets of criteria), while the remainder rated that affective symptoms predominated (which would result in a diagnosis of affective disorder with psychosis). Neither group were eager to change their rating. Indeed, it seemed that this reflected a consistent divide between the attitudes of psychiatrists on this issue. Given this fairly polarised division among clinicians, there is a likelihood of reduced reliability in diagnosing such disorders as schizoaffective disorder in classifications which do not have explicit instructions regarding their hierarchical rules.

Overcoming diagnostic problems

Linkage studies

Linkage analysis/positional cloning has produced a number of striking successes in genetic disorders, such as Duchenne's muscular dystrophy (Hoffman & Kunkel, 1989) and cystic fibrosis (Riordan *et al*, 1989). It has therefore been adopted as the main approach to the study of molecular genetics of schizophrenia. Since its instigation, linkage analysis in psychiatry has been characterised as a "bubbling cauldron of false positives" (Matthysse, 1990). For instance, Sherrington *et al* (1988) reported positive linkage between schizophrenia and a marker on chromosome 5q which has failed to be confirmed by subsequent studies (Kennedy *et al*, 1988; St Clair *et al*, 1989; McGuffin *et al*, 1990; Champion *et al*, 1992). Sherrington *et al* (1988) attempted to optimise the evidence for linkage in their study (i.e. exploring a range of test parameters ratios to achieve a set of circumstances in which the most significant result is obtained) by extending the diagnostic net to include individuals with a wide range of disorders such as mild depression or alcohol abuse. Other options include the use of alternative diagnostic systems such as changing from ICD–10 to, say, DSM–III–R if the latter produced stronger support for linkage. The obvious problem with such strategies is that of multiple testing. The greater the number of statistical comparisons undertaken within a study, the higher the likelihood of making a Type I error. Although using more than one diagnostic approach within a study can reduce its power to detect an effect, at least one is not throwing the baby out with the bathwater by being too diagnostically rigid and missing an effect. However, in adopting such a strategy one must make the appropriate statistical corrections for multiple testing (Ott, 1991) and be wary of accepting initial linkage findings, always seeking a replication of an effect before considering it to be a genuine positive result.

Following on from the above point, the choice of particular diagnostic criteria is not merely a shot in the dark. We do have indirect evidence relating to the genetic validity of some of the operational criteria. In their study of the Maudsley twin series, Gottesman & Shields (1972) found that the highest monozygotic/dizygotic concordance ratio (MZ/DZ), and therefore indirectly the 'most genetic' definition, was provided by a 'middle of the road' clinical description rather than by very broad or very narrow criteria. Subsequently, McGuffin *et al* (1984) examined the heritability of four diagnostic systems (ICD–10, Feighner, DSM–III and Schneider's First Rank Symptoms) as applied to the same Maudsley twins using OPCRIT. Broad heritabilities of approximately 84% were found for ICD–10, the Feighner criteria and DSM–III criteria. However, Schneider's First Rank Symptoms had a heritability of zero. In an expanded analysis of the DSM–III criteria where a broad range of diagnoses were applied to the twins, Farmer *et al* (1987) found that MZ/DZ was at its highest when the criteria for co-twin concordance included affective disorder with psychosis and mood-incongruent delusions, atypical psychosis and schizotypal personality as well as schizophrenia, but that further additions such as paranoid disorder, depression or any psychiatric disorder reduced MZ/DZ.

Some implications of extending the phenotype in linkage studies of schizophrenia have recently been explored using simulation techniques (Matthysse & Parnas 1992). They suggest that the recent failures to replicate reports of linkage could be due to lack of power. They demonstrate that extending the phenotype to include disorders and abnormalities which are genetically related to schizophrenia (i.e. more commonly found in relatives of schizophrenics than schizophrenia itself) substantially increased the statistical power of linkage studies. These included schizotypal personality disorder and abnormal eye movements (Kendler *et al*, 1981; Holzman, 1992). Actual linkage studies of schizophrenia have attempted to accommodate extended phenotypes by using both broad and narrow definitions of cases (Gill *et al*, 1993) and by including performance measures such as the P300 response (Blackwood *et al*, 1991).

Another solution is to examine differing phenotypic severity and adjust the analysis by specifying appropriate 'liability classes'. This is based on the notion that liability to a complex disorder is a usually unobserved variable that is continually distributed in the population (Falconer, 1965). This opens the way for using continuous measures of disease severity, which is an issue that has provoked much interest of late. The quantification of disease severity is better established in the study of affective than psychotic disorders. At the forefront of this research is the work of Rice *et al* (1986, 1992), whose detailed analysis of the diagnostic stability of major affective disorders produced combinations of signs and symptoms that could act as continuous measures of liability to have the disorder. In the case of major depressive disorder, a combination of the number of affective symptoms and treatment predicted liability. Rice went on to suggest that these increasing liability levels could be incorporated into linkage liability classes.

Association studies

In the absence of replicated positive linkage findings for psychotic disorder, recent attention has turned to studies of association. Plomin (1990) has eloquently argued that nearly all genetically influenced behaviours, whether normal or abnormal, are likely to reflect the additive effects of many genes at different loci. If many genes of minor effect do play a significant role in the aetiology of psychotic illness, then studies of association offer a viable approach to their discovery. The main method in association studies is to identify so called marker 'candidate genes', which may plausibly have a direct effect on liability to the disorder (Owen & McGuffin, 1992). Of late, the number of possible 'candidate genes' has rapidly increased. In particular, five dopamine receptor types have been identified. The dopamine D3 receptor is of especial interest in schizophrenia because of its expression in the limbic areas of the brain. The neuroleptic clozapine has been shown to have a close affinity to the D4 receptor. To date, few association studies on psychotic illness have been carried out, but their application in the future is promising. Indeed, an association between homozygosity at the D3 receptor gene and schizophrenia has been shown, but the study awaits replication (Crocq *et al*, 1992).

Small samples have insufficient power to detect minor genetic effects, and as with linkage studies, large multicentre collaborations are required. Although the problems of caseness definition are less problematic than for linkage studies, it remains imperative to collect phenotypic information carefully to ensure diagnostic unanimity between centres.

Conclusions

Psychiatric diagnosis in the field of molecular genetics research has taken something of a rollercoaster journey from problems to solutions to yet more problems. However, with the broadening of the diagnostic approach to include 'normal' behavioural dimensions and with increasing emphasis on continuous measures of disease severity, more appropriate solutions may be found. In many ways the changes in diagnostic approach reflect the changing theoretical underpinnings of the field. With research failing to support the predictions of a single gene model of schizophrenia (McGue *et al*, 1985), models postulating the co-action or interaction of major and minor genes (Risch, 1990) or minor genes (Plomin, 1990) have come to the fore. Thus a broader and more detailed account of the phenotype is necessary to meet the changing demands of molecular genetics research.

References

AMERICAN PSYCHIATRIC ASSOCIATION (1987) *Diagnostic and Statistical Manual of Mental Disorders* (3rd edn, revised) (DSM–III–R). Washington, DC: APA.

—— (1994) *Diagnostic and Statistical Manual of Mental Disorders* (4th edn) (DSM–IV). Washington, DC: APA.

BLACKWOOD, D. H. R., ST CLAIR, D. M., MUIR, W. J., *et al* (1991) Auditory P300 and eye tracking dysfunction in schizophrenic pedigrees. *Archives of General Psychiatry*, **48**, 899–909.

BROCKINGTON, I. F., KENDELL, R. E. & LEFF, J. P. (1978) Definitions of schizophrenia: concordance and prediction of outcome. *Psychological Medicine*, **8**, 387–398.

CARPENTER, W. T., STRAUSS, J. S. & BARTKO, J. J. (1973) Flexible system for the diagnosis of schizophrenia: a report from the WHO Pilot Study of Schizophrenia. *Science*, **182**, 1275.

CHAMPION, D., D'AMATO, T., LAKLOU, H., *et al* (1992) Failure to replicate linkage between chromosome 5q11–q13 markers and schizophrenia in 28 families. *Psychiatry Research*, **44**, 171–179.

CROCQ, M. A., MANT, R., ASHERSON, P., *et al* (1992) Association between schizophrenia and homozygosity at the D3 receptor gene. *Journal of Medical Genetics*, **29**, 858–860.

CROW, T. J. (1980) The molecular pathology of schizophrenia: more than one disease process? *British Medical Journal*, **280**, 66–68.

FALCONER, D. S. (1965) The inheritance of liability to certain diseases, estimated from the incidence among relatives. *Annals of Human Genetics*, **29**, 51–76.

FARMER, A. E., MCGUFFIN, P. & SPITZNAGEL, E. L. (1983) Heterogeneity in schizophrenia: a cluster analytic approach. *Psychiatry Research*, **8**, 1–12.

——, —— & GOTTESMAN, I. I. (1987) Twin concordance for DSM–III schizophrenia: scrutinizing the validity of the definition. *Archives of General Psychiatry*, **44**, 634–641.

——, WESSELY, S., CASTLE, D., *et al* (1992) Methodological issues in using a polydiagnostic approach to define psychotic illness. *British Journal of Psychiatry*, **161**, 824–831.

——, COSYNS, P., LEBOYER, R. M., *et al* (1993) A SCAN–SADS comparison study of psychotic subjects and their first degree relatives. *European Archives of Psychiatry and Clinical Neuroscience*, **242**, 352–359.

FEIGHNER, J. P., ROBINS, E., GUZE, S. B., *et al* (1972) Diagnostic criteria for use in psychiatric research. *Archives of General Psychiatry*, **26**, 57–67.

FOULDS, G. A. (1965) *Personality and Personal Illness*. London: Tavistock.

GILL, M., MCGUFFIN, P., PARFITT, E., *et al* (1993) A linkage study of schizophrenia with DNA markers from the long arm of chromosome 11. *Psychological Medicine*, **23**, 27–44.

GOTTESMAN, I. I. (1991) *Schizophrenia Genesis: The Origins of Madness*. New York: W. H. Freeman.

—— & SHIELDS, J. (1993) *Schizophrenia and Genetics: A Twin Study Vantage Point*. New York: Academic Press.

HOFFMAN, E. & KUNKEL, L. (1989) Dystrophin abnormalities in Duchenne/Becker muscular dystrophy. *Neuron*, **2**, 1019–1029.

HOLZMAN, P. S. (1992) Behavioral markers of schizophrenia useful for genetic studies. *Journal of Psychiatric Research*, **26**, 427–445.

KENDELL, R. E. (1975) *The Role of Diagnosis in Psychiatry*. Oxford: Blackwell.

KENDLER, K. S., GRUENBERG, A. M. & STRAUSS, J. S. (1981) An independent analysis of the Copenhagen sample of the Danish adoption study of schizophrenia, II: The relationship of schizotypal personality disorder and schizophrenia. *Archives of General Psychiatry*, **38**, 982–984.

KENNEDY, J. L., GIUFFRA, L. A., CAVALLI-SFORZA, L. L., *et al* (1988) Evidence against linkage of schizophrenia to markers on chromosome 5 in a northern Swedish pedigree. *Nature*, **336**, 167–170.

LEBOYER, M. & MCGUFFIN, P. (1991) Collaborative strategies in the molecular genetics of the major psychoses. *British Journal of Psychiatry*, **158**, 605–610.

MANNUZZA, S., FRYER, A. J., KLEIN, D. F., *et al* (1986) Schedule for affective disorders and schizophrenia: lifetime version modified for the study of anxiety disorders (SADS-LA). Rationale and conceptual development. *Journal of Psychiatric Research*, **20**, 317–325.

MATTHYSSE, S. (1990) Genetic linkage and complex diseases: a comment. *Genetic Epidemiology*, **7**, 29–31.

—— & PARNAS, J. (1992) Extending the phenotype of schizophrenia: implications for linkage analysis. *Journal of Psychiatric Research*, **26**, 329–344.

McGUE, M., GOTTESMAN, I. I. & RAO, D. C. (1985) Resolving genetic models for the transmission of schizophrenia. *Genetic Epidemiology*, **2**, 99–110.

McGUFFIN, P., FARMER, A. E., GOTTESMAN, I.I., *et al* (1984) Twin concordance for operational definitions of schizophrenia. *Archives of General Psychiatry*, **41**, 541–545.

——, SARGENT, M. P., HETT, G., *et al* (1990) Exclusion of a schizophrenia susceptibility gene from the 5q11–q13 region: new data and a re-analysis of previous reports. *American Journal of Human Genetics*, **47**, 524–535.

——, FARMER, A. E. & HARVEY, I. (1991) A polydiagnostic application of operational criteria in studies of psychotic illness: development and reliability of the OPCRIT system. *Archives of General Psychiatry*, **48**, 764–770.

—— MURRAY, R. M. (1991) *The New Genetics of Mental Illness*. Oxford: Heinemann.

OTT, J. (1991) *Analysis of Human Genetic Linkage* (2nd edn). Baltimore: Johns Hopkins University Press.

OWEN, M. & McGUFFIN, P. (1992) The molecular genetics of schizophrenia: blind alleys, acts of faith, and difficult science. *British Medical Journal*, **305**, 664–665.

PLOMIN, R. (1990) The role of inheritance in behaviour. *Science*, **348**, 133–138.

PULL, M. C., PULL, C. B. & PICHOT, P. (1987) Des criteres empiriques français pour les psychoses, II: consensus des psychiatres français et definitions provisories. *Encephale*, **13**, 53–57.

RICE, J. P., McDONALD-SCOTT, P., ENDICOTT, J., *et al* (1986) The stability of diagnosis with an application to bipolar II disorder. *Journal of Psychiatric Research*, **19**, 285–296.

——, ROCHBERG, N., ENDICOTT, J., *et al* (1992) Stability of psychiatric diagnoses: an application to the affective disorders. *Archives of General Psychiatry*, **49**, 824–296.

RIORDAN, J. R., ROMMENS, J. M., KEREM, B., *et al* (1989) Identification of the cystic fibrosis gene: cloning and characterization of complementary DNA. *Science*, **245**, 1066–1073.

RISCH, N. (1990) Linkage strategies for genetically complex traits: I. Multilocus models. *American Journal of Human Genetics*, **46**, 222–228.

ROBINS, L. N., WING, J., WITTCHEN, H. V., *et al* (1988) The composite international diagnostic interview. *Archives of General Psychiatry*, **45**, 1069–1078.

SCHNEIDER, K. (1959) *Clinical Psychopathology* (trans. M. Hamilton). New York: Grune & Stratton.

SHERRINGTON, R., BRYNJOLFSSON, J., PETURSSON, H., *et al* (1988) Localization of a susceptibility locus on chromosome 5. *Nature*, **336**, 164–167.

SPITZER, R. L., ENDICOTT, J. & ROBINS, E. (1975) *Research Diagnostic Criteria. Instrument No. 58*. New York: New York State Psychiatric Institute.

ST CLAIR, D., BLACKWOOD, D., MUIR, W., *et al* (1989) No linkage of chromosome 5q11–q13 markers to schizophrenia in Scottish families. *Nature*, **339**, 305–309.

STEPHENS, J. H., ASTRUP, C., CARPENTER, W., *et al* (1982) A comparison of nine systems to diagnose schizophrenia. *Psychiatry Research*, **6**, 127–143.

TAYLOR, M. A. & ABRAMS, R. (1978) The prevalence of schizophrenia: a reassessment of using modern diagnostic criteria. *American Journal of Psychiatry*, **135**, 945–948.

TSUANG, M. T. & WINOKUR, G. (1974) Criteria for subtyping schizophrenia. *Archives of General Psychiatry*, **31**, 43–47.

WING, J. F., BABOR, T., BRUGHA, J., *et al* (1990) SCAN: Schedules for Clinical Assessment in Neuropsychiatry. *Archives of General Psychiatry*, **47**, 589–593.

WORLD HEALTH ORGANIZATION (1992) *The ICD–10 Classification of Mental and Behavioural Disorders*. WHO Geneva.

Part II. Biological advances

4 Biological markers in the major psychoses

DOUGLAS H. R. BLACKWOOD and WALTER J. MUIR

Genetic studies in schizophrenia and manic–depressive illness are made difficult by the uncertain phenotype of these illnesses, diagnosed primarily by clinical interview, which may allow good reliability but cannot confer validity. There is a long-term quest for biological variables of diagnostic value, for at least some subgroups of psychotic patients, that could act as indicators of risk of illness in susceptible individuals and which could direct research towards the particular brain dysfunctions underlying these diseases. Disturbances of eye movements in 'dementia praecox' were first identified over 80 years ago (Diefendorf & Dodge, 1908) and are now one of the strongest candidates for a schizophrenic trait marker. Other biochemical and pharmacological studies have focused mainly on peripheral measures of monoamine metabolism, and the application of these to genetic studies has been well reviewed elsewhere (Goldin et al, 1987; Propping & Friedl, 1988).

This chapter will focus on alterations both in latency and amplitude of event related potentials, and on the impairment of smooth pursuit eye tracking in the psychoses. There is an increasing consensus that stable impairments of these measures occur in these illnesses. This raises the question of the utility of physiological markers in clarifying the genetic transmission of the psychoses within families, and also the relationship of these markers to abnormalities in brain structural morphology detected by imaging techniques.

Event related potentials

Abnormalities in the spontaneous electroencephalogram have long been recognised in schizophrenia (Flor-Henry et al, 1979), but the changes are non-specific. Event related potentials, particularly those generated by auditory stimuli, show more promise as biological markers on account of improved specificity and because they provide a means of monitoring cognitive processes. Used in conjunction with neuropsychological testing and brain imaging, they are a powerful tool for investigating the nature and the neuro-anatomical localisation of the brain disturbance in the psychoses.

The 'gating' involved in the processing of auditory information is thought to be defective in schizophrenic patients. One illustration of this is the failure to suppress the P50 wave of the auditory evoked potential to the second of a pair of click stimuli in a conditioning-testing paradigm. The P50 wave is a positive-going response around 50 ms post-stimulus, and when paired clicks are presented to normal subjects the P50 response to the second click is suppressed or 'gated'. The failure to gate this response has been related to the inability of some schizophrenic patients to filter competing stimuli in the environment correctly. It has been further proposed that the auditory gating deficit is secondary to hippocampal dysfunction, and represents a 'schizotaxic factor' necessary but not sufficient for the development of schizophrenia in an individual (Adler & Waldo, 1991). From the viewpoint of biological markers, it is of interest that the sensory gating abnormality was detected in approximately half of the first degree relatives, generally including at least one parent (Siegel *et al*, 1984).

The P300 event related potential

The P300 is another event related potential with several characteristics suggesting its usefulness as a schizophrenic trait marker in certain contexts. The P300 is a positive-going wave that occurs around 300 ms after an infrequently occurring stimulus to which the subject is attending. It has been subject to extensive psychological investigation and has relationships to various mental processes, including task difficulty, memory and stimulus evaluation time, justifying the term 'cognitive' event related potential. It meets several of the requirements for a biological trait marker in schizophrenia, since abnormalities of latency and/or amplitude are found in the patient population and a percentage of their relatives (Roth & Cannon, 1972; Shagass *et al*, 1977; Baribeau-Brown *et al*, 1983; Brecher & Begleiter, 1983; Pfefferbaum *et al*, 1983; Barrett *et al*, 1986; Romani *et al*, 1987; Ebmeier *et al*, 1990; McCarley *et al*, 1991; Ogura *et al*, 1991; Muir *et al*, 1991). It seems largely independent of medication effects, does not show significant sex differences and is present across the subtypes of schizophrenia (Blackwood *et al*, 1987; St Clair *et al*, 1989; Muir *et al*, 1991). Its relation to the age of the subject is well known, and it also shows test-retest reliability. Furthermore, when applied to family studies it is found that in relatives of schizophrenic patients, P300 latency is bimodally distributed (Blackwood *et al*, 1991*a*).

However, the overall validity of P300 latency and amplitude as markers is still uncertain, and it is clear that changes are not specific to schizophrenia but are found in normal ageing and in various types of dementia (Goodin *et al*, 1978; Pfefferbaum *et al*, 1983; St Clair *et al*, 1985), mental handicap, including Down's syndrome (Blackwood *et al*, 1988*b*; Muir *et al*, 1988), manic–depressive illness (Muir *et al*, 1991) and in certain groups of alcoholics and their relatives (Porjesz *et al*, 1980; Begleiter *et al*, 1984).

Recent discussions on the clinical usefulness of P300 as a diagnostic tool in dementia are also highly pertinent to schizophrenia and other psychoses. Pfefferbaum *et al* (1990) stressed the confounding effects of age, sex, medication and clinical state, which combine to make prolonged P300 latency a diagnostic marker with low sensitivity and poor specificity for dementia. The counter-argument (Goodin, 1990) is that P300 and other event related potentials are no less specific than tests such as computerised tomography (CT) and magnetic resonance imaging (MRI), which have an established place in clinical diagnosis and investigation. For example, the widespread use of the electroencephalogram (EEG) in the diagnosis of epilepsy is set against a background of 52% sensitivity and 96% specificity for the detection of epileptiform activity in the EEG of suspected epileptics. Even if P300 latency and amplitude changes are non-specific for schizophrenia and fail to distinguish schizophrenic from manic–depressive psychosis, they would still be useful in two special and important situations: firstly, in 'high risk' studies for the detection of individuals who may subsequently develop illness; and secondly, when used in conjunction with brain imaging and neuropsychological testing to investigate the underlying disorder of brain function in the psychoses.

P300 in 'high risk' studies

In a group of 45 schizophrenic probands from selected families with more than one schizophrenic member, P300 latency was found to be increased and the amplitude reduced compared with a group of 212 normal controls (Blackwood *et al*, 1991*a*). In the non-schizophrenic first and second degree relatives of these patients, a bimodal distribution of P300 latency was also found. In the 41 family members with significantly delayed latency, 18 had major psychiatric illnesses, including manic–depressive illness and schizoaffective disorder, but 19 subjects had no history of any psychiatric illness. Many of these relatives had passed the major risk period for developing schizophrenia. In a further study, a group of relatives with abnormally prolonged P300 latency were shown to have the same abnormal profile of neuropsychological test results, including impaired performance in verbal fluency testing, as found in the schizophrenic population (Roxborough *et al*, 1993). Segregation analysis of P300 latency change in this group of relatives indicated that it may be a useful measure of the genetic predisposition to schizophrenia among asymptomatic relatives, but did not support a monogenic model for the transmission of schizophrenia (Sham *et al*, 1994).

Another approach with high-risk subjects is longitudinal. For instance, the visual event-related potentials of children with a schizophrenic parent have been studied and not found different from children of normal controls (Friedman *et al*, 1988). However, Saitoh *et al* (1984), using another visual paradigm, demonstrated reduced P300 amplitude in siblings of schizophrenic patients compared with controls. Using an auditory stimulus, Schreiber *et al* (1991) examined a total of 48 children aged 7–17 years, 24 of whom were at high risk for schizophrenia, having at least one parent with the illness, and matched with the other 24 who were controls with no family history of schizophrenia. The high-risk group had significantly prolonged P300 latency and also performed poorly on psychometric tests, including those addressing reaction time, IQ and attention. A subsequent study (Schreiber *et al*, 1992), using a slightly different listening task, found a reduction of P300 amplitude that correlated significantly with psychometric deficit. Friedman *et al* (1988), however, examined symptomless adolescents at increased risk of schizophrenia and affective disorder (having an affected parent) and found that P300 recorded during an auditory task did not discriminate between the high-risk and control groups.

P300 and brain imaging

The neural origins of scalp-recorded auditory P300 responses are unknown, but several lines of evidence suggest multiple generators, including loci in the region of the auditory cortex and superior temporal and inferior parietal association areas (Lovrich *et al*, 1988; Rogers *et al*, 1991). Depth electrode recording during a two-tone discrimination task suggested that potentials generated in the medial temporal lobe structures could be a source (Halgren *et al*, 1980; Smith *et al*, 1986; Meador *et al*, 1987; Stapleton & Halgren, 1987; Richer *et al*, 1989; Smith *et al*, 1990), but they appeared to be ruled out as a primary source of P300 when Stapleton *et al* (1987) recorded normal P300 responses from 11 subjects who had undergone temporal lobectomy. Smith *et al* (1990), in a study of ten epileptic patients, concluded that the inferior parietal cortex was a major contributor to scalp-recorded P300. In patients with discrete neurological brain lesions examined by Knight *et al* (1988, 1989), auditory P300 response was impaired little by lateral parietal cortex lesions, but discrete unilateral lesions in the posterior-superior temporal plane eliminated P300 response altogether, implying that the auditory association cortex is critical for P300 generation.

A few studies have combined structural imaging with neurophysiological recording. Romani *et al* (1987) recorded auditory P300 and related this to computerised tomograms of 20 schizophrenic subjects, and found no association between ventricular enlargement and P300 latency or amplitude. However, McCarley *et al* (1989) with nine schizophrenic patients and nine controls, found that left Sylvian fissure enlargement on CT scanning significantly correlated with reduced P300 amplitude over the left temporal region. Blackwood *et al* (1991*b*), measuring several brain regions from serial coronal MRI scans of 31 schizophrenics and 33 controls, found that prolonged P300 latency in schizophrenics correlated with enlarged lateral ventricles and a reduced right and left anterior cingulate cortex area. In a further study (Blackwood *et al*, 1994), single photon emission computerised tomography (SPECT) with the intravenous blood flow marker ^{99m}Tc-exametazine was carried out in 14 acutely ill, drug-free schizophrenic patients, of whom auditory P300 was measured within a few days of scanning. P300 latency significantly correlated with tracer uptake into the left superior pre-frontal and left parietal regions, suggesting that the prolonged P300 latency of schizophrenia is a reflection of mainly left-sided frontal and temporal dysfunction. This is broadly in keeping with the view offered by McCarley *et al* (1991) that P300 amplitude reduction is mainly left sided in schizophrenia and correlates with CT changes in the left side. In a recent development of their work, McCarley *et al* (1993) have combined P300 recordings with MRI and found a significant association in 15 schizophrenic subjects between P300 amplitude reduction and volume reduction in the left posterior-superior temporal gyrus.

Eye tracking dysfunction

The ocular motility of schizophrenics has been a source of fascination for psychiatrists for a considerable length of time (Diefendorf & Dodge, 1908; Couch & Fox, 1934; White, 1938), but it was Holzman's report over twenty years ago (Holzman *et al*, 1973) of a disturbance of smooth pursuit movements that renewed the interest of biological psychiatrists. The finding that the incidence of such eye tracking dysfunction differs from a normal control population has proven to be most robust, enduring multiple independent attempts at replication (Shagass *et al*, 1974, 1976; Kuechenmeister *et al*, 1977; Pass *et al*, 1978; Cegalis & Sweeney, 1979, 1981; Iacono *et al*, 1982; Bartfai *et al*, 1983; Scarone *et al*, 1987; Blackwood *et al*, 1988*a*; Spohn *et al*, 1988). The anomaly can be described as an apparent inefficiency of the smooth pursuit system with an excess of saccadic intrusions and bursts of saccadic tracking interspersed into seemingly normal periods of smooth tracking (Levin *et al*, 1982*a*).

However, there is still controversy over the relative contributions of smooth pursuit and saccades to the abnormality. The intrinsic kinetics of the saccades themselves seem to be similar to normal controls (Iacono *et al*, 1981; Levin *et al*, 1981*a,b*, 1982*a*; Mather & Puchat, 1982/3; Done & Frith, 1984;

Yee *et al*, 1987), although in a non-pursuit task, smaller saccades have been reported (Cegalis *et al*, 1982). The locational accuracy of saccades also seems reasonably intact. If the saccades were truly intact then a decreased pursuit system gain would be suspected, and Yee *et al* (1987) have reported this but with some degree of overlap with controls. Whatever the mechanism involved, explanations based on simple inattention or lack of motivation (Brezinova & Kendell, 1977) are difficult to maintain when other types of eye tracking that do not involve the smooth pursuit system but demand an equal level of voluntary attention remain unaffected (Lipton *et al*, 1980*a,b*; Iacono *et al*, 1981; Levin *et al*, 1982*b*; Mather *et al*, 1989).

Neuroleptic medication does not seem to alter smooth pursuit performance (Shagass *et al*, 1974; Holzman, 1975; Holzman & Levy, 1977; Iacono *et al*, 1981; Muir *et al*, 1992), and the abnormality persists with remission of psychotic symptoms (Levy *et al*, 1983*a*). However, it is important to note that the most commonly used measures of eye tracking such as the signal-to-noise ratio or the r.m.s. error figures, although having the benefit of being simple to apply, may mask many differential effects. Rea *et al* (1989), for example, have reported changes in the saccades, but not pursuit, with clinical state and medication, and suggest that the former is the trait marker. Test-retest stability on the whole seems good (Lindsey *et al*, 1978; Levin *et al*, 1981*a*; Lipton *et al*, 1983). The methodological situation has been well reviewed by Clementz & Sweeney (1990).

The eye movement disorder is familial, and Holzman's findings (Holzman *et al*, 1974, 1984) that nearly 50% of schizophrenics' first degree relatives have eye tracking dysfunction (ETD), compared with around 8% of normal subjects, suggested the possible use of ETD as a genetic marker and have been broadly replicated (Kuechenmeister *et al*, 1977; Mather, 1985; Siegel *et al*, 1984). Blackwood *et al* (1991*a*) found that ETD in large schizophrenic pedigrees, like P300, had a bimodal distribution in relatives. Twin studies lend further support, and the pairwise concordance rate for ETD in monozygotic twins discordant for schizophrenia is higher than that found in dizygotics (Holzman *et al*, 1977, 1978, 1980). However, ETD does not always co-segregate with the clinical phenotype, but instead shows pleiotropy. Schizophrenics with normal eye tracking may have parents with ETD, and monozygotic twins are found with the schizophrenic having normal eye tracking and the clinically normal co-twin showing ETD (Holzman, 1987). To account for these findings, a latent trait hypothesis has been proposed, whereby an assumed single gene anomaly can phenotypically present as schizophrenia or ETD or both (Matthysse *et al*, 1986; Matthysse & Holzman, 1987; Holzman *et al*, 1988; Holzman, 1989).

The utility of ETD in psychiatric genetics is unfortunately limited by uncertainty about the specificity of dysfunction to schizophrenia. ETD has been found in major affective disorders in many studies (Shagass *et al*, 1974; Klein *et al*, 1976; Salzman *et al*, 1978; Lipton *et al*, 1980*b*;

Levin *et al*, 1981*a*; Iacono *et al*, 1982). The first degree relatives of patients with bipolar illness do not seem to show an increased rate of ETD (Levy *et al*, 1983*b*; Holzman *et al*, 1984), and Levy and her colleagues have shown that lithium therapy for bipolar illness impairs smooth pursuit (Levy *et al*, 1985). Relevant to the concept of a schizophrenia spectrum, it is of interest that patients with schizotypal personality disorder may also share the dysfunction (Keefe *et al*, 1989).

The central nervous system substrate for ETD is as yet uncertain. SPECT imaging studies suggest a relation to the frontal lobes (Blackwood *et al*, 1994), and the frontal eye fields are known to be involved in the oculomotor control of smooth pursuit. It is of interest that eye movements of patients with right frontal lobe lesions were impaired in a geometric figure visualisation task in a similar way to schizophrenics (Matsushima *et al*, 1992).

Conclusions

Changes in the P300 event related potential and eye tracking dysfunction are probably our best candidates for biological and genetic markers for major psychotic disorders. Problems still exist as to their ability to differentiate between the psychoses in general populations, but applied to the genetic study of large multiplex kindreds they could prove very useful indicators of a disordered genotype. The integration of P300 and eye movement recordings with increasingly powerful brain imaging techniques and neuropsychological testing will allow a much more detailed analysis of the dysfunctions themselves and the underlying disorder they at least partly represent.

References

ADLER, L. E. & WALDO, M. C. (1991) Counterpoint: a sensory gating hippocampal model of schizophrenia. *Schizophrenia Bulletin*, **17**, 19–24.

BARIBEAU-BROWN, J., PICTON, T. W. & GOSELIN, J. Y. (1983) Schizophrenia: a neurophysiological evaluation of abnormal information processing. *Science*, **219**, 874–876.

BARRETT, K. McCALLUM, W. C. & POCOCK, P. V. (1986) Brain indicators of altered attention and information processing in schizophrenic patients. *British Journal of Psychiatry*, **148**, 414–420.

BARTFAI, A., LEVANDER, S. E. & SEDVALL, G. (1983). Smooth pursuit eye movements, clinical symptoms, CSF metabolites, and skin conductance habituation in schizophrenia patients. *Biological Psychiatry*, **18**, 971–987.

BEGLEITER, H., PORJESZ, B., BIHARI, B., *et al* (1984) Event-related brain potentials in boys at risk for alcoholism. *Science*, **225**, 1493–1496.

BLACKWOOD, D. H. R., WHALLEY, L. J., CHRISTIE, J. E., *et al* (1987) Changes in auditory P3 event-related potential in schizophrenia and depression. *British Journal of Psychiatry*, **150**, 154–160.

——, ST CLAIR, D. M. & MUIR, W. J. (1988*a*) P300 and smooth pursuit eye tracking abnormalities in schizophrenics and their relatives. *Schizophrenia Research*, **1**, 177–178.

———, ———, ———, *et al* (1988*b*) The development of Alzheimer's disease in Down's syndrome assessed by auditory event-related potentials. *Journal of Mental Deficiency Research*, **32**, 439–453.

———, ———, ———, *et al* (1991*a*) Auditory P300 and eye tracking dysfunction in schizophrenic pedigrees. *Archives of General Psychiatry*, **48**, 899–909.

———, YOUNG, A. H., McQUEEN, J. K., *et al* (1991*b*) Magnetic resonance imaging in schizophrenia: altered brain morphology associated with P300 abnormalities and eye tracking dysfunction. *Biological Psychiatry*, **30**, 753–769.

———, EBMEIER, K. P., MUIR, W. J., *et al* (1994) Correlation of regional cerebral blood flow equivalents measured by single photon emission computerised tomography with P300 latency and eye movement abnormality in schizophrenia. *Acta Psychiatrica Scandinavica* (in press).

BRECHER, M. & BEGLEITER, H. (1983) Event-related brain potentials to high-incentive stimuli in unmedicated schizophrenic patients. *Biological Psychiatry*, **18**, 661–674.

BREZINOVA, V. & KENDELL, R. E. (1977) Smooth pursuit eye movements of schizophrenics and normal people under stress. *British Journal of Psychiatry*, **130**, 59–63.

CEGALIS, J. A. & SWEENEY, J. A. (1979) Eye movements in schizophrenia: a quantitative analysis. *Biological Psychiatry*, **14**, 13–26.

——— & ——— (1981) The effect of attention on smooth pursuit eye movements of schizophrenics. *Journal of Psychiatric Research*, **16**, 145–161.

———, ——— & DELLIS, E. M. (1982) Refixation saccades and attention in schizophrenia. *Psychiatry Research*, **7**, 189–198.

CLEMENTZ, B. A. & SWEENEY, J. A. (1990) Is eye movement dysfunction a biological marker for schizophrenia? A methodological review. *Psychological Bulletin*, **108**, 77–92.

COUCH, F. H. & FOX, J. C. (1934) Photographic study of ocular movements in mental disease. *Archives of Neurology and Psychiatry*, **34**, 556–578.

DIEFENDORF, A. R. & DODGE, R. (1908) An experimental study of the ocular reactions of the insane from photographic records. *Brain*, **31**, 451–489.

DONE, D. J. & FRITH, C. D. (1984) Automatic and strategic control of eye movements in schizophrenia. In *Theoretical and Applied Aspects of Eye Movement Research* (eds A. G. Gale & F. Johnson), pp. 481–487. Amsterdam: North Holland.

EBMEIER, K. P., POTTER, D. D., COCHRANE, R. H. B., *et al* (1990) P300 and smooth eye pursuit: concordance of abnormalities and relation to clinical features in DSM–III schizophrenia. *Acta Psychiatrica Scandinavica*, **82**, 283–288.

FLOR-HENRY, P., KOLES, Z. J., HOWARTH, B. G., *et al* (1979) Neurophysiological studies of schizophrenia, mania and depression. In *Hemisphere Asymmetries of Function in Psychopathology* (eds J. Gruzelier & P. Flor-Henry), pp. 189–222. New York: Elsevier.

FRIEDMAN, D., SUTTON, S., PUTTNAM, L., *et al* (1988) ERP components in picture matching in children and adults. *Psychophysiology*, **25**, 570–590.

GOLDIN, L. R., DE LISI, L. E. & GERSHON, E. S. (1987) Genetic aspects to the biology of schizophrenia. In *Handbook of Schizophrenia, Vol. 2. Neurochemistry and Neuropharmacology of Schizophrenia* (eds F. A. Henn & L. E. De Lisi), pp. 467–492. New York: Elsevier.

GOODIN, D. S. (1990) Clinical utility of long latency 'cognitive' event-related potentials (P3): the pros. *Electroencephalography and Clinical Neurophysiology*, **76**, 2–5.

———, SQUIRES, K. C. & STARR, A. (1978) Long latency event related components of the auditory evoked potential in dementia. *Brain*, **101**, 635–648.

HALGREN, E., SQUIRES, N. K., WILSON, C. L., *et al* (1980) Endogenous potentials generated in the human hippocampal formation and amygdala by infrequent events. *Science*, **210**, 803–805.

HOLZMAN, P. S. (1975) Smooth pursuit eye movements in schizophrenia: recent findings. In *The Biology of the Major Psychoses: A Comparative Analysis* (ed. D. X. Freedman), pp. 217–231. New York: Raven Press.

——— (1987) Recent studies of psychophysiology in schizophrenia. *Schizophrenia Bulletin*, **13**, 49–75.

——— (1989) The use of eye movement dysfunctions in exploring the genetic transmission of schizophrenia. *European Archives of Psychiatry and Clinical Neuroscience*, **239**, 43–48.

——, PROCTOR, L. R., & HUGHES, D. W. (1973) Eye-tracking patterns in schizophrenia. *Science*, **181**, 179–181.

——, ——, LEVY, D. L., *et al* (1974) Eye-tracking dysfunction in schizophrenic patients and their relatives. *Archives of General Psychiatry*, **31**, 143–151.

——, KRINGLEN, E., LEVY, D. L., *et al* (1977) Abnormal pursuit eye movements in schizophrenia. *Archives of General Psychiatry*, **34**, 802–805.

—— & LEVY, D. L. (1977) Smooth pursuit eye movements and functional psychoses: a review. *Schizophrenia Bulletin*, **3**, 15–27.

——, KRINGLEN, E., LEVY, D. L., *et al* (1978) Smooth pursuit eye movements in twins discordant for schizophrenia. *Journal of Psychiatric Research*, **14**, 111–120.

——, ——, ——, *et al* (1980) Deviant eye tracking in twins dicordant for psychosis: a replication. *Archives of General Psychiatry*, **37**, 627–631.

——, SOLOMON, C. M., LEVIN, S., *et al* (1984) Pursuit eye movement dysfunctions in schizophrenia. *Archives of General Psychiatry*, **41**, 136–139.

——, KRINGLEN, E., MATTHYSSE, S., *et al* (1988) A single dominant gene can account for eye tracking dysfunctions and schizophrenia in offspring of discordant twins. *Archives of General Psychiatry*, **45**, 641–647.

IACONO, W. G., TUASON, V. B. & JOHNSON, R. A. (1981) Dissociation of the smooth-pursuit and saccadic eye tracking in remitted schizophrenics. *Archives of General Psychiatry*, **38**, 991–996.

——, PELOQUIN, L. J., LUMRY, A. E., *et al* (1982) Eye tracking in patients with unipolar and bipolar affective disorders in remission. *Journal of Abnormal Psychology*, **91**, 35–44.

KEEFE, R. S. E., SIEVER, L. J., MOHS, R. C., *et al* (1989) Eye tracking, schizophrenic symptoms and schizotypal personality disorder. *European Archives of Psychiatry and Clinical Neuroscience*, **39**, 39–42.

KLEIN, R. H., SALZMAN, L. F., JONES, F., *et al* (1976) Eye tracking in psychiatric patients and their offspring. *Psychophysiology*, **13**, 186.

KNIGHT, R. T., SCABINI, D., WOODS, D. L., *et al* (1988) The effects of lesions of superior temporal gyrus and inferior parietal lobe on temporal and vertex components of the human AEP. *Electroencephalography and Clinical Neurophysiology*, **70**, 499–509.

——, ——, *et al* (1989) Contributions of the temperal-parietal junction to the human auditory P3. *Brain Research*, **498**, 190–194.

KUECHENMEISTER, C. A., LINTON, P. H., MUELLER, T. V., *et al* (1977) Eye tracking in relation to age, sex and illness. *Archives of General Psychiatry*, **34**, 578–579.

LEVIN, S., HOLZMAN, P. S., ROTHENBURG, S. J., *et al* (1981*a*) Saccadic eye movements in psychotic patients. *Psychiatry Research*, **5**, 47–58.

——, LIPTON, R. B. & HOLZMAN, P. S. (1981*b*) Pursuit eye movements in psychopathology: effect of target characteristics. *Biological Psychiatry*, **16**, 255–267.

——, JONES, A., STARK, L., *et al* (1982*a*) Identification of abnormal patterns in eye movements of schizophrenic patients. *Archives of General Psychiatry*, **39**, 1125–1130.

——, ——, ——, *et al* (1982*b*) Saccadic eye movements of schizophrenic patients measured by reflected light technique. *Biological Psychiatry*, **17**, 1277–1287.

LEVY, D. L., LIPTON, R. B., HOLZMAN, P. S., *et al* (1983*a*) Eye tracking dysfunction unrelated to clinical state and treatment with haloperidol. *Biological Psychiatry*, **18**, 813–819.

——, YASILLO, N. J., DORUS, E., *et al* (1983*b*) Relatives of unipolar and bipolar patients have normal pursuit. *Psychiatry Research*, **10**, 285–293.

——, DORUS, E., SHAUGHNESSY, R., *et al* (1985) Pharmacologic evidence for specificity of pursuit dysfunction to schizophrenia. *Archives of General Psychiatry*, **42**, 335–341.

LINDSEY, D. T., HOLZMAN, P. S., HABERMAN, S., *et al* (1978) Smooth-pursuit eye movements: a comparison of two measurement techniques for studying schizophrenia. *Journal of Abnormal Psychology*, **87**, 491–496.

LIPTON, R. B., FROST, L. & HOLZMAN, P. S. (1980*a*) Smooth pursuit eye movements, schizophrenia and distraction. *Perception and Motor Skills*, **50**, 159–167.

——, LEVIN, S. & HOLZMAN, P. S. (1980*b*) Horizontal and vertical pursuit eye movements, the oculocephalic reflex and the functional psychoses. *Psychiatry Research*, **3**, 193–203.

——, LEVY, D. L., HOLZMAN, P. S., *et al* (1983) Eye movement dysfunctions in psychiatric patients: a review. *Schizophrenia Bulletin*, **9**, 13–31.

LOVRICH, D., NOVIC, B. & VAUGHAN, H. G. (1988) Topographic analysis of auditory event-related potentials associated with acoustic and semantic focusing. *Electroencephalography and Clinical Neurophysiology*, **71**, 40–54.

MATHER, J. A. (1985) Eye movements of teenage children of schizophrenics: a possible inherited marker of susceptibility to the disease. *Journal of Psychiatric Research*, **19**, 523–532.

—— & PUCHAT, C. (1982/3) Motor control of schizophrenics: 1. Oculomotor control of schizophrenics: a deficit in sensory processing, not strictly in motor control. *Journal of Psychiatric Research*, **17**, 343–360.

——, NEUFELD, R. W., MERSKEY, H., *et al* (1989) Release of saccades in schizophrenics: inattention or inefficiency? *European Archives of Psychiatry and Clinical Neuroscience*, **239**, 23–26.

MATSUSHIMA, E., KOJIMA, T., OHBAYASHI, S., *et al* (1992) Exploratory eye movements in schizophrenic patients and patients with frontal lobe lesions. *European Archives of Psychiatry and Clinical Neuroscience*, **241**, 210–214.

MATTHYSSE, S., HOLZMAN, P. S. & LANGE, K. (1986) The genetic transmission of schizophrenia: application of mendelian latent structure analysis to eye tracking dysfunctions in schizophrenia and affective disorder. *Journal of Psychiatric Research*, **20**, 57–76.

—— & —— (1987) Genetic latent structure models: implications for research on schizophrenia. *Psychological Medicine*, **17**, 271–274.

MCCARLEY, R. W., FAUX, S. F., SHENTON, M., *et al* (1989) CT abnormalities in schizophrenia: a preliminary study of their correlations with P300/P200 electrophysiological features and positive/negative symptoms. *Archives of General Psychiatry*, **46**, 698–708.

——, ——, ——, *et al* (1991) Event related potentials in schizophrenia: their biological and clinical correlates and a new model of schizophrenic pathophysiology. *Schizophrenia Research*, **4**, 209–231.

——, SHENTON, M. E., O'DONNELL, B. F., *et al* (1993) Auditory P300 abnormalities and left posterior superior temporal gyrus volume reduction in schizophrenia. *Archives of General Psychiatry*, **50**, 190–197.

MEADOR, K. J., LORING, D. W., KING, D. W., *et al* (1987) Limbic evoked potentials predict site of epileptic focus. *Neurology*, **37**, 494–497.

MUIR, W. J., SQUIRE, I., BLACKWOOD, D. H. R., *et al* (1988) Auditory P300 response in the assessment of Alzheimer's disease in Down's syndrome: a two year follow-up study. *Journal of Mental Deficiency Research*, **32**, 455–463.

——, ST CLAIR, D.M. & BLACKWOOD, D. H. R. (1991) Long-latency auditory event-related potentials in schizophrenia and in bipolar and unipolar affective disorder. *Psychological Medicine*, **21**, 867–879.

——, ——, ——, *et al* (1992) Eye tracking dysfunction in the affective psychoses and schizophrenia. *Psychological Medicine*, **22**, 573–580.

OGURA, C., NAGEISHI, Y., MATSUBAYSAHI, M., *et al* (1991) Abnormalities in event-related N100, P200, P300 and slow wave in schizophrenia. *Japanese Journal of Psychiatry and Neurology*, **45**, 57–65.

PASS, H. L., SALZMAN, L. F., KLORMAN, R., *et al* (1978) The effect of distraction on acute schizophrenics' visual tracking. *Biological Psychiatry*, **13**, 587–593.

PFEFFERBAUM, A., WENEGRAT, B. G., FORD, J. M., *et al* (1983) Clinical applications of the P3 component of event-related potentials: II. Dementia, depression and schizophrenia. *Electroencephalography and Clinical Neurophysiology*, **59**, 104–124.

——, FORD, J. M. & KRAEMER, H. C. (1990) Clinical utility of long latency 'cognitive' event-related potentials (P3): the cons. *Electroencephalography and Clinical Neurophysiology*, **76**, 6–12.

PORJESZ, B., BEGLEITER, H. & SAMUELLY, I. (1980) Cognitive deficits in chronic alcoholics and elderly subjects assessed by evoked brain potentials. *Acta Psychiatrica Scandinavica*, **62** (suppl. 286), 15–29.

PROPPING, P. & FREIDL, W. (1988) Genetic studies of biochemical, pathophysiological and pharmacological factors and schizophrenia. In *Handbook of Schizophrenia, Vol. 3. Neurology, Epidemiology and Genetics* (eds M. T. Tsuang & J. C. Simpson), pp. 579–608. New York: Elsevier.

REA, M. M., SWEENEY, J. A., SOLOMON, C. M., *et al* (1989) Changes in eye tracking during clinical stabilization in schizophrenia. *Psychiatry Research*, **28**, 31–39.

RICHER, F., ALAIN, C., ACHIM, A., *et al* (1989) Intracerebral amplitude distributions of the auditory evoked potential. *Electroencephalography and Clinical Neurophysiology*, **74**, 202–208.

ROGERS, R. L., BAUMANN, S. B., PAPANICOLAU, A. C., *et al* (1991) Localization of the P3 sources using magnetoencephalography and magnetic resonance imaging. *Electroencephalography and Clinical Neurophysiology*, **79**, 308–321.

ROMANI, A., MERELLO, S., GORRELI, L., *et al* (1987) P300 and CT scan in patients with chronic schizophrenia. *British Journal of Psychiatry*, **151**, 506–513.

ROTH, W. T. & CANNON, E. (1972) Some features of the auditory evoked response in schizophrenics. *Archives of General Psychiatry*, **27**, 466–471.

ROXBOROUGH, H. M., MUIR, W. J., BLACKWOOD, D. H. R., *et al* (1993) Neuropsychological and P300 abnormalities in schizophrenics and their relatives. *Psychological Medicine*, **23**, 305–314.

ST CLAIR, D. M., BLACKWOOD, D. H. R. & CHRISTIE, J. E. (1985) P3 and other long latency auditory evoked potentials in presenile dementia, Alzheimer's type dementia and alcoholic Korsakoff syndrome. *British Journal of Psychiatry*, **147**, 702–707.

——, —— & MUIR, W. J. (1989) P300 abnormality in schizophrenic subtypes. *Journal of Psychiatric Research*, **23**, 49–55.

SAITOH, O., NIWA, S., HIRAMATSU, K., *et al* (1984) Abnormalities in late positive components of event related potentials may reflect a genetic predisposition to schizophrenia. *Biological Psychiatry*, **19**, 293–303.

SALZMAN, L. F., KLEIN, R. H. & STRAUSS, J. S. (1978) Pendulum eye tracking in remitted psychiatric patients. *Journal of Psychiatric Research*, **14**, 121–126.

SCARONE, S., GAMBINI, O., HAFELE, E., *et al* (1987) Neurofunctional assessment of schizophrenia: a preliminary investigation of the presence of eye-tracking (SPEMS) and quality extinction test (QET) abnormalities in a sample of schizophrenic patients. *Biological Psychiatry*, **24**, 253–259.

SCHREIBER, H., STOLZ-BORN, G., KORNHUBER, H. H., *et al* (1992) Event-related potential correlates of impaired selective attention in children at high risk of schizophrenia. *Biological Psychiatry*, **32**, 634–651.

——, ——, ROTHMEIER, J., *et al* (1991) Endogenous event-related brain potentials and psychometric performance in children at risk from schizophrenia. *Biological Psychiatry*, **30**, 177–189.

SEIGEL, C., WALDO, M., MIZNER, G., *et al* (1984) Deficits in sensory gating in schizophrenic patients and their relatives. *Archives of General Psychiatry*, **41**, 607–612.

SHAGASS, C., AMADEO, M. & OVERTON, D. A. (1974) Eye tracking performance in psychiatric patients. *Biological Psychiatry*, **9**, 245–260.

——, ROEMER, R. A. & AMADEO, M. (1976) Eye-tracking performance and engagement of attention. *Archives of General Psychiatry*, **33**, 121–125.

——, STRAUMANIS, J. J., ROEMER, R. A., *et al* (1977) Evoked potentials of schizophrenics in several sensory modalities. *Biological Psychiatry*, **12**, 221–231.

SHAM, P. C., MORTON, N. E., MUIR, W. J., *et al* (1994) Segregation analysis of complex phenotypes: an application to schizophrenia and auditory P300 latency. *Psychiatric Genetics*, **4**, 29–38.

SMITH, M. E., STAPLETON, J. M. & HALGREN, E. (1986) Human medial temporal lobe potentials evoked in memory and language tasks. *Electroencephalography and Clinical Neurophysiology*, **63**, 145–159.

——, HALGREN, E., SOKOLIK, M., *et al* (1990) The intracranial topography of the P3 event-related potential elicited during auditory oddball. *Electroencephalography and Clinical Neurophysiology*, **76**, 235–248.

SPOHN, H. E., COYNE, L. & SPRAY, J. (1988) The effect of neuroleptics and tardive dyskinesia on smooth-pursuit eye movement in chronic schizophrenics. *Archives of General Psychiatry*, **45**, 833–840.

STAPLETON, J. M. & HALGREN, E. (1987) Endogenous potentials evoked in simple cognitive tasks: depth components and task correlates. *Electroencephalography and Clinical Neurophysiology*, **67**, 44–52.

——, —— & MORENO, K. A. (1987) Endogenous potentials after anterior temporal lobe lobectomy. *Neuropsychologia*, **25**, 549–557.

WHITE, H. R. (1938) Ocular pursuits in normal and psychopathological subjects. *Journal of Experimental Psychology*, **22**, 17–31.

YEE, R. D., BALOGH, R. W., MARDER, S. R., *et al* (1987) Eye movements in schizophrenia. *Investigative Ophthalmology and Visual Science*, **28**, 366–374.

5 Tourette's syndrome and obsessive–compulsive behaviours

VALSAMMA EAPEN and
MARY M. ROBERTSON

Gilles de la Tourette's syndrome (GTS) is characterised by multiple motor and one or more vocal tics of more than a year's duration, and an age of onset before 21 years (American Psychiatric Association, 1987). In 1885, George Gilles de la Tourette described nine cases of GTS and suggested that it was familial. Although the hereditary nature of the disorder had been recognised from the time of its original description, only recently have attempts been made to understand the precise genetic mechanisms involved.

Earlier studies found that a higher proportion of GTS patients had a family history of GTS or of chronic motor tics (CMT) than controls (Eldridge *et al*, 1977; Shapiro *et al*, 1978; Nee *et al*, 1980).

A genetic component

In the last decade, several studies using family history data suggested the existence of a single major gene that confers susceptibility for GTS (Baron *et al*, 1981; Kidd & Paul, 1982; Comings *et al*, 1984; Devor, 1984; Price *et al*, 1984; Curtis *et al*, 1992).

There also seems to be a familial pattern to the inheritance of obsessive–compulsive disorder (OCD). Rasmussen & Tsuang (1986) reviewed the OCD literature on twins and found that, of 51 monozygotic (MZ) twin pairs where at least one twin had OCD, 32 (63%) pairs were concordant for OCD. However, as questions about the methodology have been raised and since these reports were compiled from the literature, most consisting of small numbers of twins, these concordances should be interpreted with caution. Carey & Gottesman (1981) reported on a sample of 30 twins (15 dizygotic (DZ) and 15 MZ) where at least one twin had received a diagnosis of OCD, and found higher concordance rates for MZ than for DZ twins.

Clifford *et al* (1981, 1984) carried out genetic analyses on 419 pairs of normal twins who had been given the 42-item version of the Leyton

Obsessional Inventory (LOI; Cooper, 1970). Findings suggested that genetic and specific environmental factors were important for the manifestation of OCD. They reported heritabilities of 44% for OC traits and 47% for OC symptoms. These results support those of Carey & Gottesman (1981) and suggest that genes influence the development and expression of OCD. McGuffin & Mawson (1980) reported on two identical twin pairs who were separated before the onset of symptoms, and neither were aware of the others problems. Despite this, the OC symptoms started at similar ages and followed a similar course in both pairs. The fathers in both sets of twins were compulsively neat. It is interesting to note that one of these twins had childhood tics, and two of the two pairs of identical twins with OCD described by Inouye (1965) had GTS.

Thus while genetic factors are important in the expression of OC symptoms, it is clear that these behaviours are also influenced by environmental factors. In this regard it should be noted that in all twin data reported, the concordance for MZ twins was less than 1.0 and heritability estimates were consistently less than 1.0. In addition, an analysis of OC traits in twins (Cox *et al*, 1975) showed the strong interaction between genetic and environmental factors.

The connection

Further evidence that at least some forms of OCD are genetically determined comes from the work on GTS. Pauls *et al* (1986) reported that 23% of first degree relatives of GTS probands had OCD. About 40% of them had OCD without GTS or tics, hence approximately 10% of all relatives had OCD without tics. Additional support for an association comes from the findings of Kurlan *et al* (1986), Comings & Comings (1987), Robertson & Gourdie (1990) and Robertson & Trimble (1991), who also found that a significant number of relatives of GTS patients have OCD in the absence of tics or vocalisations.

Increased rates of obsessive–compulsive behaviours (OCB) have been reported among patients with GTS (Fernando, 1967, 1976; Sim, 1969; Nee *et al*, 1980; Yaryura-Tobias *et al*, 1981; Montgomery *et al*, 1982; Frankel, 1985; Frankel *et al*, 1986; Pauls *et al*, 1986; Pitman *et al*, 1987; Comings, 1987; Grad *et al*, 1987; Robertson *et al*, 1988). However, studies varied widely in the reporting of OC symptoms, with prevalence ranging from 11–90% (Robertson, 1989). Also, specific associations have been noted between OC phenomena and other symptoms of GTS. Robertson *et al* (1988) found that 37% of 90 GTS patients reported OCB, and that this was significantly associated with coprolalia and echo phenomena. It has been shown that these symptoms vary according to the severity of GTS; for example, frequency of echolalia has been reported to be 9.3% in grade I and 48.3% in grade III

OCB. Montgomery *et al* (1982) suggested that OC symptoms were more pronounced and severe in older patients. Of 30 patients over 21 years of age with GTS, 27 patients (90%) had OCD. Therefore selective bias in obtaining patients could result in wide variations in the reported frequencies of OC symptoms in GTS.

Initial empirical studies based on clinical samples reported that 12–35% of patients with GTS also had OCB (Kelman, 1965; Fernando, 1967; Morphew & Sim, 1969). Fernando (1967) suggested that his estimates could be conservative because they were based on a review of 85 published cases in which the absence of a report of symptoms could not be equated with the absence of the symptoms. More recent studies have indicated much higher rates, with 55–80% of GTS patients having prominent OC symptoms (Yaryura-Tobias *et al*, 1981; Nee *et al*, 1982; Jagger *et al*, 1982; Stefl, 1984). Robertson *et al* (1988) found that 37% of 90 GTS patients not only reported OC behaviour but obtained higher scores than controls. Robertson & Gourdie (1990) interviewed 85 members of a multiply-affected GTS family. Fifty were diagnosed as GTS cases, with four members having only OCB. Cases and non-cases could be distinguished on the basis of OC features and the trait score of the LOI.

Despite several reports of OCB in GTS patients, there have been few studies that included a control group. Frankel *et al* (1986) examined 63 GTS patients and 41 normal controls, and found OCB in 52% of GTS patients compared with 12.2% of the controls. Comings & Comings (1987) reported OC symptoms in 45% of GTS patients compared with 8.5% of controls. In any case, if the population prevalence of OCD is taken as 2% (Robins *et al*, 1984), it seems that the prevalence of OCD in patients with GTS is much greater than that expected by chance. Robertson *et al* (1993) compared GTS patients with depressed patients and normal controls, and showed that GTS patients are disproportionately obsessional, not accounted for by depression.

In addition to the analysis reporting the clinical relationship between OCB and GTS, studies have suggested that OCB may be aetiologically related to the syndrome. A family study by Pauls *et al* (1986) suggested that GTS and OCB are genetically related. The rate of OCD among first degree relatives was significantly higher than in the general population and a control sample of adoptive relatives. The rates of GTS, CMT and OCD were the same among relatives of probands with OCD (GTS + OCD) when compared with families of probands without OCD (GTS – OCD). The frequency of OCD without GTS or CMT among first degree relatives was significantly elevated in families of both GTS + OCD and GTS – OCD probands compared with controls.

Nicolini *et al* (1991) performed segregation analysis of 24 families of OCD, CMT and GTS subjects. The segregation ratio in the normal by normal parental mating type was 0.33 (s.d. 0.16), and 0.39 (0.14) in the normal by affected parental mating type. They were not able to reject either the autosomal dominant or recessive model, but concluded that their data suggest a dominant pattern with 80% penetrance.

Chronic motor tics

Pauls *et al* (1986) examined the hypothesis that GTS and CMT are related and gave supportive statistical evidence that the two disorders have common familial origins. The patterns of illness within the families of patients were consistent with the hypothesis that CMT are a less severe form of the syndrome. Using family history data (collected through only one or two informants per family), Kidd & Pauls (1982) tested several alternative hypotheses by means of goodness of fit procedures. They were unable to reject either a polygenic inheritance or a single major locus hypothesis. However, the single locus model gave the best statistical fit for the data. A mixed model hypothesis (one specifying a single gene with polygenic modifiers) was not examined. Other investigators have reported results of genetic analyses based on family history data and give evidence for a single major gene contributing to the expression of the syndrome.

Reporting problems

Findings are inconsistent as to the precise mode of inheritance. Previous studies have shown that family history data significantly underestimate the true rate of illness among relatives, and consequently the pattern of illness within families can be affected by this reporting bias (Pauls *et al*, 1984). For example, children reporting about their relatives may not know as much about specific symptoms in their parents compared with siblings. This reporting bias is of particular concern when studying OCD, since these individuals tend to be secretive about their illness. In many instances, they will successfully hide their symptoms from family members. In addition, some of these studies used large GTS multigenerational kindreds. These need to be interpreted with the knowledge that the bias in such multiplex families cannot easily be incorporated into the analysis. A much better test of genetic transmission can be accomplished with a large sample of small families that have been ascertained without regard to familial loading.

A recent study

Eapen *et al* (1993) performed complex segregation analysis on a sample of 40 GTS families in which all available relatives (*n* = 168) were personally interviewed. The data were analysed using the unified model as implemented in the computer program POINTER (Lalouel *et al*, 1983). POINTER has five major parameters: q is the frequency of a putative major gene; d is the degree of dominance; h is the heritability which measures background polygenic inheritance; t measures the major gene effect as the distance between two homozygotes; and τ is the transmission probability of the risk allele from heterozygous genotype. Analyses were carried out for five different diagnostic schemes; GTS only; GTS or CMT; GTS, CMT or transient tic disorder (TTD); GTS or OCB; and GTS, CMT, TTD or OCB. To incorporate age and sex differences into analyses, separate estimates of prevalence were made. For the first three diagnostic schemes, four age classes (0–5, 6–10, 11–15 and over 15) were defined for males and females separately. For the analyses that included OCB, four age classes (0–15, 16–25, 26–35 and over 35) were used. Furthermore, analyses were carried out using a wide range of population prevalences. An ascertainment probability[1] of $\pi = 0.01$ based on the method of sampling was also incorporated into the analyses. The best method for establishing a genetic relationship between GTS and OCB would involve comparing the segregation patterns observed within families when members have OCB alone (no GTS) with the patterns observed when members *are* considered to be affected by GTS.

Likelihood ratios

All hypotheses were tested using likelihood ratios. Firstly, the no-transmission model was compared with a mixed model hypothesis. Since there was evidence for vertical transmission in these families, additional analyses were performed to test specific genetic hypotheses. The generalised single locus model converged to the dominant model for all diagnostic hierarchies. For the GTS-only scheme, the mixed model solution gave parameter estimates which were almost identical to the best fitting Mendelian major locus model ($d = 1$; $t = 5.36$; $q = 0.0002$; $h = 0$; and 0% phenocopies for males and females). The mixed model moved to a boundary with the polygenic heritability (h) being zero, thus supporting the model of no polygenic heritability and rejecting the polygenic hypothesis. There was no evidence to suggest non-Mendelian transmission probabilities. For this scheme, the penetrance for males was 0.966 and females 0.452. When the definition of 'affected' status included those with GTS or OCB, the results were still consistent with an autosomal dominant model. The penetrance estimated for

---

1. The ascertainment probability, π, is the likelihood of a given individual being ascertained (sampled) for the study. Assuming there are 25 000 GTS patients in the UK and around 250 are likely to attend the GTS clinic, this gives a probability of 1% ($\pi = 0.01$). However, the analyses were repeated using different values for π, and this did not change the results or the inference.

this analysis was 0.882 for males and for females. When subjects with GTS, tics (CMT/TTD) or OCB were included, the penetrance rate was 0.980 for both sexes. As a consequence of hypothesis testing procedures under the unified model of segregation analysis, the probability of ascertainment bias due to the pedigree extension rule was considered and different values were ascribed. Changing the value of π to 0.50 and 0.99 had only negligible effect on the parameter estimates and changed none of the statistical inferences.

Goodness of fit

The goodness of fit tests (Table 5.1) were carried out for all solutions obtained for all diagnostic schemes. First degree relatives (FDRs) were grouped based on sex of the proband, sex of the relative and relationship to the proband (parents v. siblings). Expected risks of being affected with GTS, tics or OCB were calculated using the parameters of the autosomal dominant model (best fitting model) and compared with the observed rates for all FDRs using the χ^2 goodness of fit test. For the GTS-only scheme, it was noted that, when the values were estimated adequately, they predicted the observed frequencies of GTS among relatives (χ^2 with 6 degrees of freedom = 12.4; $0.05 < P < 0.10$). For the GTS or CMT group, the fit was statistically significant ($\chi^2 = 20.33$; $P < 0.005$). Similar findings were obtained when TTD was included in the above group ($\chi^2 = 21.60$; $P < 0.005$), indicating a poor fit for the data. In the GTS/OCB scheme, the fit was not statistically significant ($\chi^2 = 3.7934$; $0.9990 < P < 0.9995$) suggesting that OCB is an integral part of the spectrum of expression of the GTS syndrome. However, the GTS, CMT/TTD or OCB group gave statistically significant values ($\chi^2 = 119.465$; $P < 0.0005$), again indicating a poor fit for the data.

Results

Thus the Eapen *et al* (1993) study shows that GTS is inherited as an autosomal dominant trait with high penetrance. Furthermore, the results are consistent with the hypothesis that OCB is part of the spectrum of the

TABLE 5.1
Goodness of fit test results for all diagnostic schemes

Diagnostic scheme	χ^2	P
GTS only	12.4	$0.05 < P < 0.10$
GTS/CMT	20.3	$P < 0.005$
GTS/CMT/TTD	21.0	$P < 0.005$
GTS/OCB	3.8	$0.990 < P < 0.9995$
GTS/CMT/TTD/OCB	119.5	$P < 0.0005$

GTS = Gilles de la Tourette's syndrome, CMT = chronic motor tics, TTD = transient tic disorder, OCB = obsessive–compulsive behaviours.

syndrome. When the goodness of fit test was applied, the best fit was obtained when OCB was also included and assuming an even sex ratio. Presence of sex-dependent differences in the underlying liability was also demonstrated in this study. In order to allow comparison with previous studies, data were reanalysed using higher prevalence rates as assumed by Comings *et al* (1986) and Devor (1984), and these did not alter the inferences. Even when only those relatives with GTS were included in the analysis, the findings were consistent with autosomal dominant transmission. Although segregation analysis suggested an autosomal dominant mode of transmission for all the diagnostic schemes, the estimated values did not correspond with the observed rates in the relatives for those schemes including CMT and TTD. This suggests that some individuals with CMT do not have a form related to GTS, and that within these families, motor tics (chronic and transient) are phenocopies.

Future research

The next step in understanding the genetics of GTS will be to try to establish a linkage relationship between a marker and the hypothetical gene for the disorder. In this endeavour, it is crucial to have accurate estimates of the genetic model factors for incorporation into analysis of linkage. Studies of linkage have shown that a slight change of genetic model factors can cause large fluctuations in the results. Therefore, every attempt should be made to define the clinical phenotypes. Phenomenological studies using personal interview techniques are indicated, addressing different possible expressions of the syndrome in members of families with GTS. Questions also remain as to whether OC symptoms seen in GTS probands and relatives are different from those in OCD probands and relatives, and whether the apparent sex differences seen in GTS families are also present in OCD families.

To help understand the relationship between GTS, OCB and CMT, sound epidemiological studies are needed, particularly addressing issues such as the true estimate of GTS in the general population, and sex ratio and sex dependent differences in the expression of the disorder.

The results from the studies already mentioned do not, however, suggest that all subjects with OCD have a disorder that is aetiologically related to GTS. Recent work suggests that patients with OCD may be divided into at least two groups: those with a family history of GTS, and those without such a history (Green & Pitman, 1986). It may well be that the OC symptoms observed in members of families with GTS is a somewhat milder form, although the range and character of symptoms may or may not be different from those observed in clinical patients with OCD in the absence of GTS. George *et al* (1992) found that while violent, sexual and symmetrical obsessions, as well as forced touching, counting and self-damaging compulsions, were more common in comorbid OCD/GTS subjects, obsessions concerning dirt or germs and cleaning compulsions were more commonly encountered in OCD subjects. It remains to be seen whether the OCD which is unrelated to GTS is also familial, and, if so, whether the patterns within families are consistent with genetic transmission. The answer to questions such as how many genes are involved and what percentage of them are the GTS genes will have to await the development of a genetic marker for the GTS gene.

References

AMERICAN PSYCHIATRIC ASSOCIATION (1987) *Diagnostic and Statistical Manual of Mental Disorders* (3rd edn, revised) (DSM–III–R). Washington, DC: APA.

BARON, M., SHAPIRO, E., SHAPIRO, A., *et al* (1981) Genetic analysis of Tourette syndrome suggesting major gene effect. *American Journal of Human Genetics*, **33**, 767–775.

CAREY, G. & GOTTESMAN, I. I. (1981) Twin and family studies of anxiety, phobic and obsessive disorders. In *Anxiety: New Research and Changing Concepts* (eds D. F. Klein & J. Rabkin), pp. 117–136. New York: Raven Press

CLIFFORD, C. A., FULKER, D. W. & MURRAY, R. M. (1981) A genetic and environmental analysis of obsessionality in normal twins. In *Twin Research 3: Part B, Intelligence, Personality and Development* (ed. L. Gedda), pp. 163–168. New York: Alan Liss.

——, MURRAY, R. M. & FULKER, D. W. (1984) Genetic and environmental influences on obsessional traits and symptoms. *Psychological Medicine*, **14**, 791–800.

COMINGS, D. E., COMINGS, B. G., DEVOR, E. J., *et al* (1984) Detection of major gene for Gilles da la Tourette syndrome. *American Journal of Human Genetics*, **36**, 586–600.

——, ——, DIETZ, G., *et al* (1986) Evidence the Tourette syndrome is at 18q22.1. *Abstracts, 7th International Congress of Human Genetics*, Berlin (1986), Abstract M, 11, 23, p. 620.

—— & —— (1987) Hereditary agoraphobia and obsessive compulsive behaviour in relatives of patients with Gilles de la Tourette's syndrome. *British Journal of Psychiatry*, **151**, 195–199.

COOPER, J. (1970) The Leyton Obsessional Inventory. *Psychological Medicine*, **1**, 48–64.

COX, A., RUTTER, M., NEWMAN, S., *et al* (1975) A comparative study of infantile autism and specific developmental receptive language disorder. II: Parental characteristics. *British Journal of Psychiatry*, **126**, 146–159.

CUMMINGS, J. L. & FRANKEL, M. (1985) Gilles de la Tourette syndrome and the neurological basis of obsessions and compulsions. *Biological Psychiatry*, **20**, 1117–1126.

CURTIS, D., ROBERTSON, M. M. & GURLING, H. M. D. (1992) Autosomal dominant gene transmission in a large kindred with Gilles de la Tourette's syndrome. *British Journal of Psychiatry*, **160**, 845–849.

DEVOR, E. J. (1984) Complex segregation analysis of Gilles de la Tourette syndrome: further evidence for a major locus transmission. *American Journal of Human Genetics*, **36**, 704–709.

EAPEN, V., PAULS, D. L. & ROBERTSON, M. M. (1993) Evidence for autosomal dominant transmission in Gilles de la Tourette syndrome: United Kindom cohort study. *British Journal of Psychiatry*, **162**, 593–596.

ELDRIDGE, R., SWEET, R., LAKE, C. R., *et al* (1977) Gilles de la Tourette syndrome: clinical aspects in 21 selected families. *Neurology*, **27**, 115–124.

FERNANDO, S. J. M. (1967) Gilles de la Tourette syndrome: a report on four cases and a review of published case reports. *British Journal of Psychiatry*, **113**, 607–617.

—— (1976) Six cases of Gilles de la Tourette's syndrome. *British Journal of Psychiatry*, **128**, 436–441.

FRANKEL, M., CUMMINGS, J. L., ROBERTSON, M. M., *et al* (1986) Obsessions and compulsions in Gilles de la Tourette's syndrome. *Neurology*, **36**, 378–382.

GEORGE, M. S., TRIMBLE, M. R., RING, H. A., *et al* (1992) Obsessions in obsessive-compulsive disorder with and without Gilles de la Tourette's syndrome. *American Journal of Psychiatry*, **150**, 93–96.

GRAD, L. R., BELCOWITZ, D., OLSON, M., *et al* (1987) Obsessive compulsive symptomatology in children with Tourette's syndrome. *Journal of American Academy of Child and Adolescent Psychiatry*, **26**, 69–73.

GREEN, R. C. & PITMAN, R. K. (1986) Tourette syndrome and obsessive–compulsive disorder. In *Obsessive Compulsive Disorders: Theory and Management* (eds M. A. Jenike, L. Baer & W. O. Minichiello). Littleton, MA: PSGP.

INOUYE, E. (1965) Similar and dissimilar manifestations of obsessive compulsive neurosis in monozygotic twins. *American Journal of Psychiatry*, **121**, 1171–1175.

JAGGER, J., PRUSOFF, B. A., COHEN, D. J., *et al* (1982) The epidemiology of Tourette's syndrome: a pilot study. *Schizophrenia Bulletin*, **8**, 267–278.

KELMAN, D. H. (1965) Gilles de la Tourette's disease in children: a review of the literature. *Journal of Child Psychology and Psychiatry*, **6**, 219–226.

KIDD, K. K. & PAULS, D. L. (1982) Genetic hypothesis for Tourette syndrome. In *Gilles de la Tourette Syndrome* (eds T. N. Chase & A. J. Friedhoff) New York: Raven Press. *Advances in Neurology*, **35**, 243–249.

KURLAN, R., BEHR, J., MEDVED, L., *et al* (1986) Familial Tourette's syndrome: report of a large pedigree and potential for linkage analysis. *Neurology*, **36**, 772–776.

LALOUEL, J. M., RAO, D. C., MORTON, N. E., *et al* (1983) A unified model for segregation analysis. *American Journal of Human Genetics*, **35**, 816–826.

MCGUFFIN, P. & MAWSON, D. (1980) Obsessive compulsive neurosis: two identical twin pairs. *British Journal of Psychiatry*, **137**, 285–287.

MONTGOMERY, M. A., CLAYTON, P. J. & FRIEDHOFF, A. J. (1982) Psychiatric illness in Tourette syndrome patients and first degree relatives. In *Gilles de la Tourette Syndrome* (eds T. N. Chase & A. J. Friedhoff). New York: Raven Press. *Advances in Neurology*, **35**, 335–339.

MORPHEW, J. A. & SIM, M. (1969) Gilles de la Tourette's syndrome: a clinical and psychopathological study. *British Journal of Medical Psychology*, **42**, 293–301.

NEE, L. E., POLINSKY, R. J. & EBERT, M. H. (1980) Tourette syndrome: clinical and family studies. In *Gilles de la Tourette* (eds T. N. Chase & A. J. Friedhoff) New York: Raven Press. *Advances in Neurology*, **35**, 291–295.

NICOLINI, H., HANNA, G., BAXTER, L., *et al* (1991) Segregation analysis of obsessive compulsive and associated disorders: preliminary results. *Ursus Medicus*, **1**, 25–28.

PAULS, D. L., KRUGER, S. D., LECKMAN, J. F., *et al* (1984) The risk of Tourette's syndrome and chronic multiple tics among relatives of Tourette's syndrome patients obtained by direct interview. *Journal of American Academy of Child Psychiatry*, **23**, 134–137.

——, TOWBIN, K. E. & LECKMAN, J. F. (1986) Gilles de la Tourette syndrome and obsessive–compulsive disorder: evidence supporting a genetic relationship. *Archives of General Psychiatry*, **43**, 1180–1182.

PITMAN, R. K., GREEN, R. C., JENIKE, M. A., *et al* (1987) Clinical comparison of Tourette's disorder and obsessive compulsive disorder. *American Journal of Psychiatry*, **144**, 1166–1171.

PRICE, R. A., PAULS, D. L. & CAINE, E. D. (1984) Pedigree and segregation analysis of clinically defined subgroups of Tourette syndrome. *American Journal of Human Genetics*, (Suppl. 4), 1785.

RASMUSSEN, S. A. & TSUANG, M. T. (1986) Clinical characteristics and family history in DSM–III obsessive–compulsive disorder. *American Journal of Psychiatry*, **143**, 317–322.

ROBERTSON, M. M. (1989) The Gilles de la Tourette syndrome: the current status. *British Journal of Psychiatry*, **154**, 147–169.

——, TRIMBLE, M. R. & LEES, A. J. (1988) The psychopathology of the Gilles de la Tourette Syndrome: a phenomenological analysis. *British Journal of Psychiatry*, **152**, 383–390.

—— & GOURDIE, A. (1990) Familial Tourette's syndrome in a large British pedigree. Associated psychopathology, severity, and potential for linkage analysis. *British Journal of Psychiatry*, **156**, 515–521.

—— & TRIMBLE, M. R. (1991) Gilles de la Tourette syndrome in the Middle East: report of a cohort and a multiply affected large pedigree. *British Journal of Psychiatry*, **158**, 416–419.

———, CHANNON, S., BAKER, J., *et al* (1993) The psychopathology of Gilles de la Tourette syndrome: a controlled study. *British Journal of Psychiatry*, **162**, 114–117.

ROBINS, L. N., HELZER, J. E., WEISSMAN, M., *et al* (1984) Lifetime prevalence of specific psychiatric disorders in three sites. *Archives of General Psychiatry*, **41**, 949–958.

SHAPIRO, A. K., SHAPIRO, E. S., BRUUN, R. D., *et al* (1978) *Gilles de la Tourette Syndrome*. New York: Raven Press.

STEFL, M. E. (1984) Mental health needs associated with Tourette syndrome. *American Journal of Public Health*, **74**, 1310–1313.

YARYURA-TOBIAS, J. A., NEZIROGLU, F., HOWARD, S., *et al* (1981) Clinical aspects of Gilles de la Tourette syndrome. *Orthomolecular Psychiatry*, **10**, 263–268.

Part III. Biological treatments

6 Long-term pharmacotherapy for depression

VINCENT F. CAILLARD

Depression is no longer considered a simple episodic disease. After the recognition of the first symptoms, most patients have a long-lasting course. The episode itself may last from some weeks to some years (Keller *et al*, 1982*a*, *b*), and previous data summarised by Klerman (1978) show that if effective treatment is prematurely terminated, a relapse is observed within one year of withdrawal in at least 50–60% of cases. The same author showed that after the initial recovery, the recurrence of disease was very frequent (50–80%) in many longitudinal studies.

This high rate of recurrence is confirmed in recent prospective longitudinal studies (Lee & Murray, 1988; Kiloh *et al*, 1988), which demonstrate that after an episode, no more than 20% of patients remain free of recurrences during an 18-year follow-up period. Furthermore, depression may be a lethal disease (in these studies the risk of suicide is approximately 1 in 10) and may also evolve to chronicity in 10–20% of patients.

Two features of depression which are of considerable concern are its underrecognition and its undertreatment. This last aspect is well known, and has been recently illustrated by a drug utilisation review (McCombs *et al*, 1990); the authors reviewed all prescriptions of antidepressants made under the Medicaid scheme during a four year period in California. They found 3664 prescriptions corresponding to possible depression therapy. In 2344 cases, a minimum of one year of post-episode data were available and were analysed. The rate of consistent treatment for a major depressive episode, successful or not, was very low, with 84% of treatments considered inadequate. It is possible that in a small proportion of cases, treatment was prescribed for problems other than major depression, but most of the treatments were prescribed in subtherapeutic doses. Many patients had prematurely terminated therapy, or were noncompliant for a variety of reasons, with side-effects probably a frequent cause. A very conservative conclusion is that fewer than 25% of depressed patients receive a minimum antidepressant dose of 75 mg of imipramine or equivalent for a recommended minimum treatment period of six months.

This poses a double problem of compliance: compliance of the prescribers with established guidelines for antidepressant therapy, and patient compliance with treatment. Patient compliance is a problem which is frequently underestimated in out-patients. The noncompliance rate, even in research settings, is very high for imipramine-type antidepressants (Frank & Kupfer, 1986), averaging 50%. The rate might be reduced to an acceptable level in settings where additional psychological therapy is established.

In summary, the therapeutic strategy for this potentially chronic, disabling and lethal disorder should be considered in the long term and globally, focusing not only on the alleviation of symptoms, but also on the general acceptance of the treatment, in the setting and for the individual concerned.

Definitions

Recently, a critical review of published data during a two-year period in the most major international psychiatric journals reveals significant inconsistencies across studies in labelling the outcome of depression (Prien *et al*, 1991). Subsequently, a set of consensus definitions of terms related to outcome in recurrent depression have been proposed (Frank *et al*, 1991).

The long-term phases of the treatment are summarised in Fig. 6.1. The distinctions between remission and recovery, relapse and recurrence, are important, as they distinguish between continuation therapy and preventive therapy.

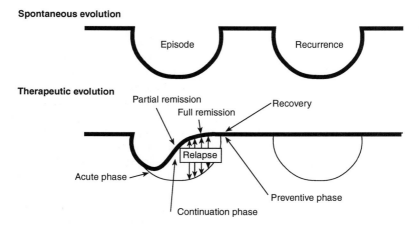

Fig. 6.1. Evolution and treatment of recurrent depression

Remission may be partial or complete. Partial remission corresponds to the alleviation of the syndrome. Some symptoms may persist, but they are in insufficient number to fulfil the syndromal definition, or their intensity may be significantly diminished. Full remission corresponds to the first no-symptoms period.

There is a widely held opinion that antidepressants act symptomatically, without modification of the hypothetical underlying depressive process. If the patient remains asymptomatic after cessation of treatment, the remission may be qualified as recovery, but this is seldomly observed in practice. Because the duration of the depressive episode is not precisely determined for any particular patient, one speaks of probable recovery after a stable period of complete remission of 4–6 months. Accordingly, one speaks of relapse when faced with reappearance or worsening of depressive symptoms occurring during this remission period. One speaks of recurrence if a new episode occurs after the 4 to 6 month remission period.

The treatment of the episode itself can be divided into acute treatment and continuation treatment. If we consider the results of controlled studies, acute treatment is not as effective as is desirable. In the vast majority of acute controlled studies, the average final score of the treated patients is close to 15 on the Hamilton depression scale after 6–8 weeks of treatment, and this is far from asymptomatic.

Thus, the acute phase of therapy attenuates the symptoms, and a crucial phase is the period of continuation therapy, the aim of which is to complete and to maintain the remission. In patients with recurrent depression, this phase must be followed by a longer-term treatment for prevention.

Continuation treatment

First generation antidepressants

The results of continuation treatment observed in controlled studies using various agents are summarised in Table 6.1, where first generation antidepressants (amitriptyline, imipramine, phenelzine and lithium) were compared with placebo in studies involving small numbers of patients over periods of 6–12 months. Most of these comparisons were made immediately after acute treatment for depression, and were designed before 1980, when precise criteria for remission and recovery did not exist. Some more recent studies were thoroughly designed, including a symptom-free period before entering double-blind study (Prien *et al*, 1984; Frank *et al*, 1990; Robinson *et al*, 1991), and outcome criteria. Early evaluation of outcome in these prophylactic studies demonstrated that amitriptyline, imipramine and phenelzine were consistently superior to placebo in the prevention of relapses.

TABLE 6.1
Controlled studies on relapse prevention

Authors	Treatments (patients)	Duration (months)	Result (% relapsed)
Amitriptyline (AMI)			
Kay *et al* (1970)	AMI/DZP 34/51	7	AMI > DZP 24% v. 47%
Mindham *et al* (1973)	AMI/P 34/27	6	AMI > P 24% v. 67%
Klerman *et al* (1974)	AMI/P 39/67	8	AMI > P 15% v. 40%
Coppen *et al* (1978)	AMI/P 13/16	12	AMI > P 0 v. 31%
Stein *et al* (1980)	AMI/P 27/28	6	AMI > P 28% v. 69%
Bialos *et al* (1982)	AMI/P 10/7	6	AMI > P 0 v. 80%
Imipramine (IMI)			
Seager & Bird (1962)	IMI/P 13/16	6	IMI > P 25% v. 69%
Mindham *et al* (1973)	IMI/P 16/15	6	IMI = P 19% v. 20%
Prien *et al* (1973)	IMI/P 25/26	4	IMI > P 32% v. 73%
Prien *et al* (1984), Greenhouse *et al* (1991)	IMI/P 41/34	(2) + 4	IMI > P 16% v. 40%
Frank *et al* (1990)	IMI/P 28/23	(6) + 6	IMI > P 18% v. 55%
Phenelzine (Phen)			
Davidson & Raft (1984)	High v. low dose 7/8	5	Hi > Lo 14% v. 100%
Robinson *et al* (1991)	Phen/P 31/16	(4) + 3	Phen > P 13% v. 75%
Lithium (Li)			
Prien *et al* (1973)	Li/P 27/25	4	Li > P 30% v. 73%
Prien *et al* (1984), Greenhouse *et al* (1991)	Li/P 37/34	(2) + 4	Li = P 37% v. 40%
Noradrenergic antidepressants			
Lendresse *et al* (1984)	NOMI/P 71/72	6	NOMI > P 20% v. 40%
Rouillon *et al* (1991)	MA75/MA37/P 385/382/375	12	MA75 > MA37 > P 16% v. 24% v. 34%
Serotoninergic antidepressants			
Doogan & Caillard (1988, 1992)	SER/P 184/106	5	SER > P 15% v. 48%
Montgomery *et al* (1988)	FLUOX/P 88/94	(4,5) + 3	FLUOX > P 13.6% v. 27.5%
Eric *et al* (1991)	PARO/P 68/67	4	PARO > P 6% v. 20%
Montgomery & Rasmussen (1991)	CIT40/CIT20/P 57/48/42	6	CIT40 ≈ CIT20 > P 13% v. 8% v. 31%

P = placebo, DZP = diazepam, NOMI = nomifensine, MA = maprotiline, SER = sertraline, FLUOX = fluoxetine, PARO = paroxetine, CIT = citalopram.

The data on lithium are obtained from two studies (Prien *et al*, 1973, 1984, revisited by Greenhouse *et al*, 1991). There is a discrepancy regarding the results, and the more recent study suggests that after effective therapy, lithium alone could be ineffective in continuation therapy. If confirmed, this is important since in some cases of poor tolerance of the acute treatment, one could be tempted to substitute lithium or to stop the antidepressant medication early under the mistaken impression that a patient undergoing lithium treatment is protected from relapse.

More recently, maintenance studies have been performed with antidepressants acting specifically on catecholamine reuptake (Lendresse *et al*, 1984; Rouillon *et al*, 1991) and on serotonin reuptake (Doogan & Caillard, 1988, 1992; Montgomery *et al*, 1988; Eric *et al*, 1991; Montgomery & Rasmussen, 1991). Those studies are also summarised in Table 6.1.

Catecholaminergic antidepressants

Studies of continuation therapy have been conducted with nomifensine and with maprotiline. Both active drugs were significantly protective against relapse. The significant difference was found in spite of a high placebo-response rate, which was probably due to the large number of neurotic depression patients included (Lendresse *et al*, 1984).

The maprotiline study (Rouillon *et al*, 1991) is very important in many aspects, especially the suggestion of a specific suicidogenic effect of maprotiline, but is also atypical and very difficult to compare with other data obtained with imipramine-like drugs. The population of patients had a mixture of major depression and dysthymic disorders (45%). They had a very high response rate (80%) with moderate doses of maprotiline (75–150 mg daily), and there was also a high response rate to placebo and to very small doses of maprotiline.

This probably relates to the very stringent definition of relapse adopted in this study, requiring a minimum score of 25 in two successive ratings of the Montgomery and Åsberg Depression Rating Scale, or a score of 27 at one examination, this score being superior even to the inclusion criterion for acute treatment, which was 25.

In spite of or because of these peculiarities, this study provides evidence for a dose–response relationship in the prevention of complete relapses, 75 mg daily being superior to 37.5 mg daily, and so on.

Selective serotonin reuptake inhibitors (SSRIs)

The results obtained with different SSRIs are concordant (see Table 6.1). A rather high placebo response rate was recorded in the fluoxetine, paroxetine and citalopram studies, though not in the sertraline study. Again, this was due to stringent criteria for relapses in these studies, where

TABLE 6.2
Controlled studies on recurrence prevention

Authors	Treatments (patients)	Duration (month)	Result (% recurr.)
First generation antidepressants			
Georgotas *et al* (1989)	PHE/NOR/P 15/13/23	(4) + 12	PHE > NOR = P 13% v. 54–65%
Robinson *et al* (1991)	PHE/P 25/26	(4) + 24	PHE > P 29% v. 81%
Prien *et al* (1973, 1984)	IMI/P 25/26 39/34	(2) + 24 (2) + 24	IMI > P 56% v. 91% 26% v. 71%
Frank *et al* (1990)	IMI/P 28/23	(6) + 36	IMI > P 21% v. 78%
Lithium (Li)			
Prien *et al* (1973)	Li/IMI/P 27/25/26	24	Li = IMI > P 63/56% v. 92%
Kane *et al* (1982)	IMI-Li/Li/IMI/P 8/7/6/6	24	IMI-Li = Li > IMI = P 13/28% v. 66/100%
Glen *et al* (1984)	Li/AMI/P 7/12/9	36	Li = AMI > P 41/57% v. 88%
Prien *et al* (1984), Greenhouse *et al* (1991)	IMI-Li/Li/IMI/P 38/37/39/34	24	IMI-Li = IMI > Li = P 26/25% > 68/71%
Selective serotonin reuptake inhibitors			
Bjork (1983)	ZIM/P 19/19	(4) + 12	ZIM > P 32% v. 84%
Doogan & Caillard (1988, 1992)	SER/P 184/106	12	SER > P 37% v. 62%
Montgomery *et al* (1988)	FLUOX/P 88/94	(6) + 12	FLUOX > P 26% v. 57%
Eric *et al* (1991)	PARO/P 68/67	12	PARO > P 15% v. 39%

P = placebo, PHE = phenelzine, NOR = nortriptyline, IMI = imipramine, ZIM = zimeldine, SER = sertraline, FLUOX = fluoxetine, PARO = paroxetine.

subsyndromal relapses were not recorded. In the sertraline study, a more naturalistic criterion using the Clinical Global Impression Scale (Guy, 1976) resulted in a more realistic evaluation of relapses. In spite of these methodological differences, all the active drugs were highly effective over the follow-up period considered.

Preventive treatment

The results of studies involving classical antidepressants, either phenelzine or imipramine, are summarised in Table 6.2. In spite of the small size of the patient groups, phenelzine and imipramine proved highly effective. Thanks to the thorough methodology, which included a symptom-free interval of 2–6 months before entering the studies, it is possible to conclude

TABLE 6.3
Summarised results on prevention of relapse and recurrence in recurrent depression

Treatment	Duration	Drug effect	Placebo effect
Relapse prevention			
antidepressants	4–12 months	82%	47%
lithium (Li)	4 months	66%	43%
noradrenergics	6–12 months	80%	63%
SSRI	4–6 months	88%	68%
Recurrence prevention			
imipramine (IMI)	2–3 years	61%	13%
lithium	2–3 years	50%	12%
IMI + Li	2 years	80%	15%
IMI + psychotherapy	3 years	76%	22%
SSRI	1 year	72%	39%

that these drugs are also effective in preventing new episodes of depression. A minimum duration of one year (up to three years of follow-up) allows a good estimate of the recurrence rate. We have no information on other first generation antidepressants, though the inefficacy of nortriptyline, observed in a small study in the elderly (Georgotas *et al* 1989), needs to be confirmed.

The data obtained for lithium (Table 6.2) suggest that in association with imipramine it may be effective in the prevention of recurrences. Lithium alone may also be effective (Prien *et al* 1973; Glen *et al*, 1984), but the more recent study (Prien *et al*, 1984; Greenhouse *et al*, 1991), as mentioned earlier, is unfortunately flawed by a high rate of early relapses.

The data on SSRIs are concordant (Montgomery & Montgomery, 1992). The methodology varied in the different studies. The use of a symptom-free period demonstrates a prevention of recurrences (Montgomery *et al* 1988), even in small studies (Bjork, 1983). Other studies obtain the same results with adequate statistical methodology using survival analysis (Doogan & Caillard, 1988, 1992; Eric *et al*, 1991). The samples studied were somewhat different, at least with regard to the placebo response rate, and this may reflect different inclusion criteria and/or different outcome criteria.

Pooling these data (Table 6.3) gives an estimation of drug efficacy in the prevention of relapses compared with no pharmacotherapy. First generation antidepressants (imipramine and phenelzine) and SSRIs are effective in the prevention of relapses as well as recurrences. Data on lithium alone are not completely convincing, due to methodological problems. Combining imipramine with lithium or with interpersonal psychotherapy may increase the response rate.

In considering dosage strategy, the maintenance dose is commonly thought to be somewhat lower than the dose needed for acute treatment, with the exception of the Pittsburgh study, or when using phenelzine. The optimal preventive doses have not been well determined. For imipramine, the Pittsburgh study (Frank *et al*, 1990) suggests that maintaining more than 200 mg of imipramine daily during three years is superior to mean doses of less than 150 mg (Prien *et al*, 1984). There is, however, no direct comparison, and in view of the toxicity of imipramine and the side-effects, which affect compliance in general practice, this claim should not be accepted without discussion. More recently, Kupfer & Frank (1992) reported that treatment with high doses of imipramine could be continued for up to five years.

For phenelzine, the optimal dose is probably equal to or greater than 45 mg daily (Robinson *et al*, 1991).

For SSRIs, unfortunately, the optimal acute effective dosage is not determined. It is therefore not surprising that guidelines for the continuation dosage or for the preventive phase cannot be given with certainty for any SSRIs. For example, the recommended acute dose of fluoxetine is now 20 mg daily, and it is suggested that even lower doses could be effective. At the time that long-term studies on fluoxetine were designed, its potency was underestimated, and although the fluoxetine study has a very stringent methodology for the demonstration of efficacy of high doses (40 to 80 mg daily), it gives no information on the standard dose for maintenance and preventive therapy in usual clinical settings.

Conclusions

Acute treatment of depression with any drug is effective in 60% of cases. In remitted patients, continuation therapy prevents relapses in 75% of cases. In recovered patients, preventive treatment for two to three years with the same agent, at the dose that was effective in acute treatment, prevents recurrences in 60% of patients at risk, and maybe more if lithium is added or if psychotherapy is associated. This demonstrates that the evolution of the depressed patient, even when adequately treated, is far from simple.

Furthermore, the results of therapy, expressed using conventional criteria, are probably too optimistic. In the short term, clinical studies show that a degree of remission is usually obtained after some weeks. In most studies, the therapeutic results are expressed in terms of the average final score of the Hamilton depression rating scale, which is not closely representative of the core symptoms of depression. In other studies, the results are expressed as a percentage of reduction of the initial score. The results demonstrate differences in the compared treatments. However, results are not always of clinical pertinence, and their meaning is obscured by the inconsistent definition of remission and recovery. In the long term, and in the majority of the studies summarised, the results are not expressed in terms of quality of remission, but in terms of prevention of the reappearance of a full syndromal definition of disease.

This methodology obscures the importance of partial remission (subsyndromal morbidity or residual symptoms) or, conversely, partial relapse and its consequences for the quality of life of treated patients and on their long-term outcome. A rigorous definition of partial remission or partial relapse is needed, since the persistence of symptoms following acute therapy may have various causes (Maj *et al*, 1992). It may be important to try to distinguish problems directly related to the depressive process and to antidepressant efficacy from those arising from other psychological or biological mechanisms, such as comorbid anxiety, anticipatory or post-traumatic anxiety. Side-effects may also sometimes be confused with depressive symptoms. Incomplete recovery from the index episode is a risk factor for subsequent relapses within one year (Favarelli *et al*, 1986).

To complete the operational criteria for relapse and remission proposed by Frank *et al* (1990), explicit criteria for subsyndromal depressive episode are also needed. They should include the core criteria for depression, with a minimum and a maximum of secondary depressive symptoms. A minimum period of stable dysphoria is required, possibly two weeks. Quantitative data should be monitored for clinical congruency, but they are of secondary importance to the fulfilment of explicit diagnostic criteria.

As far as the general conditions of therapy are concerned, optimal effective treatment is seldom achieved, mainly because of the side-effects of the reference tricyclic drugs.

The development of new selective antidepressants, which are thought to be as effective as older ones and are better tolerated, has great potential, but have these new drugs been studied as thoroughly as they should be? Their efficacy in core depression has not been as well established. There is a great need to reach a consensus on the comparative efficacy of the new selective antidepressants. Unfortunately, this aspect has not always been adequately addressed in early studies. The relative efficacy of SSRIs versus placebo in core depression needs further investigation, and dose–response relationships still need to be established for all drugs in biological depression. Thus regulatory agencies are reluctant to adopt new reference drugs with regards to efficacy, although the majority of recent drugs are better tolerated than first generation antidepressants.

The major progress in antidepressant therapy now is in improved tolerance compared with reference drugs. Further progress in efficacy will only be possible if we adopt new reference treatments that are both effective and acceptable, for the short-term treatment of depression as well as for the long term.

References

BIALOS, D., GILLER, E., JATLOW, P., *et al* (1982) Recurrence of depression after discontinuation of long-term amitriptyline treatment. *American Journal of Psychiatry*, **139**, 325–328.

BJORK, K. (1983) The efficacy of zimeldine in preventing depressive episodes in recurrent major depressive disorders – a double-blind placebo-controlled study. *Acta Psychiatrica Scandinavica*, **68** (suppl. 308), 182–189.

COPPEN, A., GHOSE, K., MONTGOMERY, S., *et al* (1978) Continuation therapy with amitriptyline in depression. *British Journal of Psychiatry*, **133**, 28–33.

DAVIDSON, J. & RAFT, D. (1984) Use of phenelzine in continuation therapy. *Neuropsychobiology*, **11**, 191–194.

DOOGAN, D. P. & CAILLARD, V. (1988) Sertraline in the prevention of relapse in major depression. *Psychopharmacology*, **96** (suppl.), 271.

——— & ——— (1992) Sertraline in the prevention of depression. *British Journal of Psychiatry*, **160**, 217–222.

ERIC, L., PETROVIC, D., LOGA, S., *et al* (1991) A prospective, double-blind, multicentre study of paroxetine and placebo in preventing recurrent major depressive episodes. Presented at World Congress of Biological Psychiatry, Florence.

FAVARELLI, C.C., AMBONETTI, A., PALLANTI, S., *et al* (1986) Depressive relapses and incomplete recovery from index episode. *American Journal of Psychiatry*, **143**, 888–891.

FRANK, E. & KUPFER, D. J. (1986) Psychotherapeutic approaches to treatment of recurrent unipolar depression: work in progress. *Psychopharmacology Bulletin*, **22**, 558–563.

———, ———, PEREL, J. M., *et al* (1990) Three-year outcomes for maintenance therapies in current depression. *Archives of General Psychiatry*, **47**, 1093–1099.

———, PRIEN, R. F., JARRETT, R. B., *et al* (1991) Conceptualization and rationale for consensus definitions of terms in major depressive disorder. Remission, recovery, relapse and recurrence. *Archives of General Psychiatry*, **48**, 851–855.

GEORGOTAS, A., McCUE, R. E. & COOPER, T. B. (1989) A placebo-controlled comparison of nortriptyline and phenelzine in maintenance therapy of elderly depressed patients. *Archives of General Psychiatry*, **46**, 783–786.

GLEN, A. I. M., JOHNSON, A. L. & SHEPHERD, M. (1984) Continuation therapy with lithium and amitriptyline in unipolar depressive illness: a randomised, double-blind controlled trial. *Psychological Medicine*, **14**, 37–50.

GREENHOUSE, J. B., SANGL, D., KUPFER, D. J., *et al* (1991) Methodologic issues in maintenance therapy clinical trials. *Archives of General Psychiatry*, **48**, 313–318.

KANE, J. M., QUITKIN, F. M., RIFKIN, A., *et al* (1982) Lithium carbonate and imipramine in the prophylaxis of unipolar and bipolar II illness. A prospective, placebo-controlled comparison. *Archives of General Psychiatry*, **39**, 1065–1069.

KAY, D. W. K., FAHY, T. & GARSIDE, R. F. (1970) A seven-month double-blind trial of amitriptyline and diazepam in ECT-treated depressed patients. *British Journal of Psychiatry*, **117**, 667–671.

KELLER, M. F., SHAPIRO, R. W., LAVORI, P. W., *et al* (1982*a*) Recovery in major depressive disorder. Analysis with the life table and regression models. *Archives of General Psychiatry*, **39**, 905–910.

———, ———, ———, *et al* (1982*b*) Relapse in major depressive disorder. Analysis with the life table. *Archives of General Psychiatry*, **39**, 911–915.

KILOH, L. G., ANDREWS, G. & NEILSON, M. (1988) The long-term outcome of depressive illness. *British Journal of Psychiatry*, **153**, 752–757.

KLERMAN, G. L. (1978) Long-term treatment of affective disorders. In *Psychopharmacology: a Generation of Progress* (ed. M. A. Lipton *et al*), pp. 1303–1311. New York: Raven Press.

———, DI MASCIO, A., WEISSMAN, M. M., *et al* (1974) Treatment of depression with drugs and psychotherapy. *American Journal of Psychiatry*, **131**, 186–191.

KUPFER, D. J. & FRANK, E. (1992) Long-term management of mood disorders. 18th collegium internationale neuro-psychopharmacologicum. Strategies, problems and implications of long-term trials on depression. *Clinical Neuropharmacology*, **15** (suppl. 1), 446A–447A.

LEE, A. S. & MURRAY, R. M. (1988) The long-term outcome of Maudsley depressives. *British Journal of Psychiatry*, **153**, 741–751.

LENDRESSE, P., CREN, M. C. & LEMARIE, J. C. (1984) Traitement prolongé par ALIVAL 75 mg dans les états dépressifs néurotiques et réactionnels. Résultats d'une étude multicentrique en double aveugle. *Psychiatrie Française*, **16**, 156–158.

MAJ, M., VELTRO, F., PIROZZI, R., *et al* (1992) Pattern of recurrence of illness after recovery from an episode of major depression: a prospective study. *American Journal of Psychiatry*, **149**, 795–800.

McCOMBS, J. S., NICHOL, M. B., STIMMEL, G. L., *et al* (1990) The cost of antidepressant drug therapy failure: a study of antidepressant use patterns in a medicaid population. *Journal of Clinical Psychiatry*, **51** (suppl. 6), 60–69.

MINDHAM, R. H. S., HOWLAND, C. & SHEPHERD, M. (1973) An evaluation of continuation therapy with tricyclic antidepressants in depressive illness. *Psychological Medicine*, **3**, 5–17.

MONTGOMERY, S. A., DUFOUR, H., BRION, S., *et al* (1988) The prophylactic efficacy of fluoxetine in unipolar depression. *British Journal of Psychiatry*, **153**, 69–76.

—— & RASMUSSEN, J. G. C. (1991) Citalopram 20 mg, citalopram 40 mg and placebo in the prevention of relapse of major depression. *International Clinical Psychopharmacology*, **6** (suppl. 5), 71–73.

—— & MONTGOMERY, D. B. (1992) Prophylactic treatment in recurrent unipolar depression. In *Long-term Treatment of Depression* (eds S. A. Montgomery & F. Rouillon). London: John Wiley & Sons.

PRIEN, R. F., KLETT, C. J. & CAFFEY, E. M. (1973) Lithium carbonate and imipramine in prevention of affective episodes. A comparison in recurrent affective illness. *Archives of General Psychiatry*, **29**, 420–425.

——, KUPFER, D. J., MANSKY, P. A., *et al* (1984) Drug therapy in the prevention of recurrence in unipolar and bipolar affective disorders. Report of the NIMH collaborative study group comparing lithium carbonate, imipramine, and a lithium carbonate-imipramine combination. *Archives of General Psychiatry*, **41**, 1096–1104.

——, CARPENTER, L. L. & KUPFER, D. J. (1991) The definition and operational criteria for treatment outcome of major depressive disorder. A review of the current research literature. *Archives of General Psychiatry*, **48**, 796–800.

ROBINSON, D. S., LERFALD, S. C., BENNETT, B., *et al* (1991) Maintenance therapies in recurrent depression new findings. *Psychopharmacology Bulletin*, **27**, 31–39.

ROUILLON, F., SERRURIER, D., MILLER, H. D., *et al* (1991) Prophylatic efficacy of maprotiline on unipolar depression relapse. *Journal of Clinical Psychiatry*, **52**, 423–431.

SEAGER, C. P. & BIRD, R. L. (1962) Imipramine with electrical treatment in depression – a controlled trial. *Journal of Mental Science*, **108**, 704–707.

STEIN, M. K., RICKELS, K. & WEISE, C. C. (1980) Maintenance therapy with amitriptyline: a controlled trial. *American Journal of Psychiatry*, **137**, 370–371.

7 Refractory depression

CORNELIUS L. E. KATONA

This chapter examines the concept and prevalence of refractory depression before focusing on the evaluation of recent evidence on possible pharmacological treatment options.

Refractory depression is a common problem in psychiatric practice. Only 60–70% of depressed patients respond to the first antidepressant drug administered to them, although a further 10–15% may improve following a course of electroconvulsive therapy (ECT) or an alternative antidepressant. Thus up to 20% of patients are treatment-refractory (Leonard, 1988). Up to 20% of all patients with depression are still depressed two years after onset (Keller *et al*, 1984).

Definition of refractory depression

Inconsistency in definition has bedevilled research into refractory depression. Remick (1989) has highlighted the importance of defining criteria for severity of illness (both at onset and following treatment) and for establishing whether prior (and apparently unsuccessful) treatment was adequately given. He further suggests that treatment resistance needs to be distinguished from inadequate prophylaxis following recovery. The concept of 'double depression', in which major depression may respond to treatment, but nonetheless leave a residual dysthymic disorder (Keller & Shapiro, 1985) adds further to the difficulties of definition.

Remick (1989) has proposed a pragmatic definition of treatment-resistant depression as "an ongoing and remitting depressed state in a patient as defined by his/her physician and who has been unsuccessfully treated with at least two different antidepressants or an antidepressant and/or course of ECT". A more operationalised approach is suggested by Nierenberg & Amsterdam (1990), with poor response to treatment defined in terms of a decrease in Hamilton Rating Scale for Depression (HRSD; Hamilton, 1967) score of less than 50% and/or a post treatment HRSD score of greater than 7.

Evaluation of treatment resistance

Guscott & Grof (1991) pointed out that a distinction needs to be made between relative and absolute treatment resistance. The crucial variables to be considered in making this distinction relate to the processes of diagnosis and treatment, rather than patient-centred variables. They identify six questions (Table 7.1) that should be considered in patients thought to be treatment-refractory.

It should not be taken for granted that the diagnosis of depression is correct in all apparently refractory patients. Even where the diagnosis is not in doubt, previous treatment must be reviewed systematically. The main foci in such a review should be dosage, duration and compliance. In patients who have made a transient response, adequacy of relapse prevention should be examined. The possible role of physical or psychosocial maintenance factors should also be considered. Some of these issues are discussed in more detail below.

Adequate dosage

An adequate dose of a tricyclic antidepressant can be defined in practical terms as the maximum tolerated dose. This will usually be associated with definite but tolerable side-effects. Such clinical dose titration has been shown to be effective in several studies (Simpson *et al*, 1976; Keller *et al*, 1982). It should be remembered that much higher doses of tricyclic antidepressants are used routinely in the USA than in the UK, in part reflecting the greater legal restraints in the USA against the use of ECT. In view of the very wide variability in plasma levels attained for a given dose, tricyclic level monitoring, if available, may also be helpful in achieving optimal dosing. This is particularly clear for imipramine, desipramine and nortriptyline (American Psychiatric Association Task Force, 1985).

TABLE 7.1
Questions to consider in evaluating treatment-resistance

1. Is the diagnosis correct?
2. Has past treatment been adequate?
3. Was a 'stepped-care' approach used?
4. How was outcome measured?
5. Is a coexistent disorder interfering with treatment response?
6. Is the clinical setting interfering with treatment response?

Adapted from Guscott & Grof (1991).

The same clinical considerations of titration to maximum tolerated dose apply for monoamine oxidase inhibitors (MAOIs) (Pare, 1985). For the relatively newly introduced selective-serotonin reuptake inhibitors (SSRIs), the value of dose titration is less clear. Indeed, Schweizer *et al* (1990) have shown that increasing the dose of the SSRI fluoxetine from 20 mg to 60 mg after three weeks in non-responders was not associated with any greater response over the next five weeks than maintenance on the original 20 mg.

Adequate duration

As the experience with fluoxetine referred to above illustrates, patients often respond to antidepressants much more slowly than the conventionally taught "three to six weeks". Greenhouse *et al* (1987) found that whereas only a quarter of their depressed subjects had responded to high dose imipramine within five weeks, half had done so by ten weeks and three-quarters by 17 weeks. Similarly, in a study of elderly depressed patients, Georgotas *et al* (1989) found that response to phenelzine and nortriptyline continued to emerge for as long as 12 weeks.

Compliance

Patient compliance should never be taken for granted. Patients (and to slightly lesser extent primary care physicians and psychiatrists) expect a rapid response to treatment. Patients experiencing a rapid onset of side-effects but no improvement for weeks on end in their depressive symptoms are acting quite reasonably in discontinuing treatment. Appropriate counselling of patients, judicious selection of antidepressants to avoid those side-effects most likely to be troublesome, and careful tablet monitoring can all contribute to the minimisation of compliance-related apparent treatment resistance.

Maintenance factors

The presence or emergence of any psychosocial maintenance factors needs thorough evaluation. These may include unrecognised physical illness, intolerable social circumstances, or secondary gain from chronic illness. Occult endocrine dysfunction may be particularly relevant in this context. Gewirtz *et al* (1988) have demonstrated occult thyroid dysfunction (manifest as elevated thyrotropin levels or low metabolic rates) in 6 out of 15 women with refractory depression, all of whom responded to thyroid supplementation. In contrast, Joffe *et al* (1992) point out that antidepressant treatment induces significant falls in thyroid hormone levels. In an open study of seven depressed patients who had failed at least three adequate antidepressant trials, they administered low doses of the antithyroid drug methimazole with the aim of reducing thyroid hormone levels while maintaining them in the normal range. Six of the subjects were able to complete the trial; three responded fully in terms of a reduction of at least 50% in HRSD score, and a further two had a partial response.

Murphy *et al* (1991) used a similar approach starting from the well-established clinical observation that hypercortisolaemia is frequently found in depression. They used a variety of steroid-suppressant drugs in an open study of ten depressed patients who had failed at least two adequate antidepressant trials. Eight of them completed the trial, of whom six responded (HRSD score reduction of at least 50%) and the other two improved significantly. The utility of careful evaluation of endocrine function in treatment-refractory depression, and the role of hormonally-based treatments clearly deserves more thorough evaluation.

Prediction of treatment resistance

Irrespective of definition, poor treatment response and chronicity within depression are predicted by a number of clinical features. Magni *et al* (1988) reported that poor response to ECT was associated with illness prior to treatment lasting for at least six months, few recent life events, and evidence of complicating physical illness. Chronicity of illness was also found to predict poor response by Schweizer *et al* (1990). Delusional depression also appears to carry a particularly poor prognosis (Murphy, 1983; Roose *et al*, 1983) and subjects with abnormalities of personality, particularly high neuroticism, can also be expected to do badly (Duggan *et al*, 1990).

Pharmacological strategies

A variety of treatments, including ECT (Fink, 1989) and psychosurgery (Malizia, this volume) are effective in refractory depression. Most clinicians, as shown in two recent surveys, favour the use of pharmacological strategies. Nierenberg (1991) described a case vignette (of a 40-year-old female in-patient with DSM–III–R major depression failing to respond to four weeks of treatment with nortriptyline) to psychiatrists in the US attending educational meetings on refractory depression. The most popular strategy among the psychiatrists was the addition of lithium (34%), followed by continuing the nortriptyline for a further two weeks (only 18%, reflecting the lack of appreciation of the frequent occurrence of late response to antidepressants), switching to an SSRI (16%), ECT (11%) and switching to an MAOI (7%). In contrast, the most popular manoeuvres in cases of non-response to tricyclics reported by a sample of Canadian psychiatrists (Chaimowitz *et al*, 1991) were giving an MAOI (22%) and adding lithium (19%).

Evidence for the utility of combinations of antidepressants, with each other or with other psychoactive drugs, and on the use of MAOIs and SSRIs as sole agents, will be evaluated in this chapter. It must be emphasised that most reports lack adequate placebo-control and are not carried out specifically in refractory patients. Emphasis will be placed on formal clinical trials (blind and open-label) rather than case reports, and on evidence specifically obtained in refractory patients. Several novel treatment manoeuvres, focusing mainly on enhancing serotonergic or noradrenergic neurotransmission, have been proposed. These are summarised in Table 7.2, but have only received very little formal evaluation and (with the exception of the hormonal therapies referred to earlier) are not described here in any detail.

Single agents

Monoamine oxidase inhibitors (MAOIs)

The use of MAOIs in refractory depression has been supported by both open and double-blind clinical trials, although the total number of evaluated patients remains small. In an open trial of 47 subjects with major depression treated unsuccessfully with at least two antidepressants, Nolen *et al* (1988) found tranylcypromine to be affective for 50% of the patients. Response was particularly good in those with endogenous depressions of relatively short duration. Similarly, Georgotas *et al* (1983) reported that 65% of a cohort of elderly treatment-resistant depressives responded to phenelzine.

Thase *et al* (1992*a*) gave a six-week open-label trial of MAOIs (predominantly tranylcypromine) to 42 patients who had failed to respond to a combination of imipramine and interpersonal psychotherapy, and reported a response rate of 58%. Response was significantly higher in the subgroup with anergic atypical depression. The same group (Thase *et al*, 1992*b*) reported on 16 patients with bipolar depression whose treatment had

TABLE 7.2
Novel pharmacological strategies in refractory depression

Manoeuvre	Reference
Thyroid suppression	Joffe *et al*, 1992
Adrenocortical suppression	Murphy *et al*, 1991
Reserpine augmentation	Price *et al*, 1987
Yohimbine augmentation	Schmauss *et al*, 1988*a*
Fenfluramine augmentation	Price *et al*, 1990
Buspirone augmentation	Bakish, 1991
Fluoxetine augmentation	Weilburg *et al*, 1989
Carbamazepine	Cullen *et al*, 1991
Psychostimulant augmentation	Fawcett *et al*, 1991
Combined SSRI and tricyclics	Seth *et al*, 1992
Bright-light augmentation	Levitt *et al*, 1991
Vanadium ion inactivation	Kay *et al*, 1984

been crossed over to the other drug (maintaining the blind) following failure to respond in a controlled comparison between imipramine and tranylcypromine. Nine of the 12 imipramine non-responders recovered on tranylcypromine, in contrast with only one of the four tranylcypromine non-responders doing well when switched to imipramine. Very similar results have been reported by McGrath *et al* (1993) in a series of patients with non-melancholic depression. Those failing to respond during an initial double-blind comparison between phenelzine and imipramine were crossed over (maintaining the blind) to the other drug. Subsequent response was 67% in the group switched to phenelzine, but only 41% of phenelzine non-responders recovered on imipramine.

Serotonin selective reuptake inhibitors

Preliminary evidence suggests that fluoxetine and fluvoxamine are effective in non-responders to other antidepressants. In an extensive open study of response to fluoxetine in subjects failing to respond to imipramine, amitriptyline or doxepin, Beasley *et al* (1990) reported that between 51% and 62% of subjects responded to fluoxetine, the exact response rate depending on the rigour with which treatment resistance was defined. Delgado *et al* (1988) reported that eight (29%) out of 28 subjects with refractory depression responded to 4–6 weeks of open fluvoxamine. Similarly, in a small but double-blind crossover to fluvoxamine (White *et al*, 1990) in 12 desipramine non-responders, nine (75%) improved, although only four (33%) recovered completely.

Drug combinations

Monoamine reuptake inhibitor (MARI) and MAOI

Although initial reports of severe adverse effects have been made for this combination, more recent studies have suggested that concurrent administration at relatively low doses renders it relatively safe (Razani *et al*, 1983; Pare, 1985). Controlled clinical trials (which were not carried out for treatment-refractory patients) suggest that MARI + MAOI is not superior to treatment with a single antidepressant. Schmauss *et al* (1988*b*), however, carried out a retrospective analysis of 94 patients with refractory depression treated with tranylcypromine in combination with tricyclic or tetracyclic antidepressants, and found a 68% response rate with a good side-effect profile.

MARI and tri-iodothyronine

Open studies (Earle, 1970; Goodwin *et al*, 1982) demonstrated marked improvement after the addition of tri-iodothyronine for 22 out of 37 patients, mainly female, who had been unresponsive to tricyclics alone. A small double-blind controlled study by Wheatley (1972) showed superiority of response after 10 and 14 days in patients treated with amitriptyline and tri-iodothyronine compared with those on amitriptyline alone. However, the patients were not selected for treatment resistance, only low doses of amitriptyline were used, and the duration of the trial was inadequate to assess whether response was merely hastened.

A more recent open study of adjunctive tri-iodothyronine in imipramine-resistant recurrent depression (Thase *et al*, 1989*a*), following the same methods as their other trials with lithium augmentation (Thase *et al*, 1989*b*) and MAOIs (Thase *et al*, 1992*a*,*b*), found a response rate of only 25% following the addition of tri-iodothyronine. This was no different to the response rate in a historical comparison group receiving continued tricyclics alone.

L-tryptophan

L-tryptophan may be a useful adjunct to MAOIs, and possibly to tricyclic antidepressant treatment. Coppen *et al* (1963) reported that tranylcypromine and L-tryptophan in combination resulted in a clearly superior outcome compared with tranylcypromine alone in a double-blind controlled trial. Similar potentiation of clomipramine by L-tryptophan was reported by Walinder *et al* (1976), although the duration of the trial was short, the plasma clomipramine levels were higher in the combination treated group, and the patients were not selected for treatment-resistance.

These results were not confirmed by a study combining L-tryptophan with the SSRI zimelidine (Walinder *et al*, 1981). L-tryptophan may nonetheless be a useful adjunct in refractory depression. It has been suggested that its efficacy in augmenting antidepressant response may be enhanced by the co-administration of allopurinol, to prevent metabolism of the L-tryptophan along the kyneurenine rather than the serotonin pathway targeted by the therapy (Shopsin, 1978). L-tryptophan is now only available in the UK on a named-patient basis, following reports of an eosinophilia–myalgia syndrome. It is, however, almost certain that the syndrome resulted from a contaminant (Eccleston *et al*, 1991).

Tricyclic–neuroleptic combinations

Depressive illness complicated by delusions or hallucinations is associated with poor response to antidepressants, and carries a poor prognosis (Glassman *et al*, 1975). The literature review by Spiker *et al* (1985) confirmed that response to tricyclics alone was as low as 34%, and to major tranquillisers alone, 48%. Studies of the combination of major tranquilliser and tricyclic, however, showed an overall response rate as high as 81%. The studies reviewed were open and their diagnostic criteria variable. Spiker *et al* (1985) attempted to confirm the findings in a small double-blind controlled comparison between amitriptyline alone, perphenazine alone and the combination. Although response to each of the drugs alone was low (19% to perphenazine alone and 41% to amitriptyline alone), 78% responded to the combination, a figure comparable to what might be expected from ECT (Janicak *et al*, 1985). The combination of major tranquilliser and tricyclic antidepressant may thus be a useful alternative to ECT in delusional depression, although the results might in part reflect the fact that major tranquillisers increase plasma tricyclic levels (Spiker *et al*, 1986).

Lithium augmentation

De Montigny *et al* (1981) reported a dramatic response within 48 hours to the addition of lithium in patients who had not responded to at least three weeks of treatment with tricyclic antidepressants. The efficacy of the combination, although not the rapidity of the response, has since been confirmed in a large number of case reports and open trials (reviewed by Katona, 1988), and in a rather smaller number of patients treated under double-blind placebo-controlled conditions. The open trials reviewed by Katona (1988) found that, of a total of 219 patients evaluated, 53% showed clinically adequate responses and a further 12% partial responses. Since the publication of that review, at least seven further studies (Delgado *et al*, 1988; Dinan & Barry, 1989; Thase *et al*, 1989*b*; Dallal *et al*, 1990; Ontiveros *et al*, 1991; Zimmer *et al*, 1991; Rybakowski & Matkowski, 1992) have been published, and the total number of patients treated with lithium in open studies stands at 406. Response rate in the augmented sample is hardly altered, with 54% response and 9% partial response.

A very wide variety of antidepressants was used before lithium augmentation. Ontiveros *et al* (1991) reported that response to lithium augmentation in patients treated with fluoxetine tended to be faster than those treated with desipramine, but the relapse rate was higher in the fluoxetine group. Rybakowski & Matkowski (1992), however, failed to identify particular antidepressants associated with higher or lower likelihood of response. They did find that satisfactory response to lithium augmentation was associated with less severe depression, and with the emergence of partial response within the first week following administration of lithium.

The results of six small double-blind controlled trials of lithium augmentation (Heninger *et al*, 1983; Cournoyer *et al*, 1984; Kantor *et al*, 1986; Zusky *et al*, 1988; Schopf *et al*, 1989; Stein & Bernadt, 1993) in a total of 111 patients have been subjected to a meta-analysis by Austin *et al* (1991). Although interpretation of the data is made difficult by the variable duration of exposure to lithium and the inclusion, in the Stein & Bernadt (1993) study, of a 'low-dose' lithium group, the results are broadly in keeping with the results of the open studies. They show a clear and statistically significant superiority for lithium augmentation over continued antidepressant alone, and provide considerable support for the widely held clinical view that lithium augmentation is a useful treatment option.

The mechanism of lithium's augmentatory action remains unclear. Blier & De Montigny (1985) suggested that lithium enhances 5HT neurotransmission. Support for this comes from the findings by Cowen *et al* (1989) that lithium enhances the prolactin response to L-tryptophan in depressed patients. Cowen *et al* (1991), however, failed to demonstrate any difference in this response between those subjects with refractory depression who responded to lithium augmentation and those who did not. They concluded that their results provided only limited support for the hypothesis that changes in brain 5HT function are involved in the antidepressant response to lithium augmentation. The variable onset of antidepressant response to lithium augmentation also fails to resolve whether the critical response is a true augmentation, a synergism or simply the antidepressant effect that is well documented for lithium alone (Worrall *et al*, 1979).

Of greater relevance is the fact that lithium augmentation may be effective where other strategies such as tri-iodothyrodine augmentation have failed (Garbutt *et al*, 1986); indeed, the combination of lithium and tranylcypromine may succeed even where lithium augmentation of other antidepressants has failed (Price *et al*, 1985).

An important unresolved clinical issue is the further drug management of patients who have responded to lithium augmentation. The only study of this issue to date (Nierenberg *et al*, 1990) found that, of 66 patients followed-up for a mean of 29 months after attempted lithium augmentation, 48% had good outcomes and a further 23% a fair outcome. The only predictor of good outcome was good initial response; neither continuation of antidepressant nor continuation of lithium was significantly associated with outcome.

Conclusions

It is clear from this brief review that lithium augmentation and the use of MAOIs (in that order) are at present the best supported pharmacological strategies for refractory depression. Several other 'rational' strategies show some promise, but require adequate placebo-controlled evaluation. Full re-evaluation of apparently refractory patients is vital before embarking on any refractory treatment regime. The question of prophylaxis in refractory patients who finally respond has hardly been addressed so far. It is clear, however, that pharmacological strategies have the potential to improve very considerably the outlook for that considerable proportion of patients who fail to respond to first-line antidepressant treatment.

References

AMERICAN PSYCHIATRIC ASSOCIATION TASK FORCE (1985) Tricyclic antidepressants – blood level measurements and clinical outcome: an APA task force report. *American Journal of Psychiatry*, **142**, 155–162.

AUSTIN, M. P. V., SOUZA, F. G. M. & GOODWIN, G. M. (1991) Lithium augmentation in antidepressant-resistant patients. A quantitative analysis. *British Journal of Psychiatry*, **159**, 510–514.

BAKISH, D. (1991) Fluoxetine potentiation by buspirone: three case histories. *Canadian Journal of Psychiatry*, **36**, 749–750.

BEASLEY, C. M., SAYLER, M. E., CUNNINGHAM, G. E., et al (1990) Fluoxetine in tricyclic-refractory major depressive disorder. *Journal of Affective Disorders*, **20**, 193–200.

BLIER, P. & DE MONTIGNY, C. (1985) Short-term lithium administration enhances serotonergic neurotransmission: electrophysiological evidence in the rat CNS. *European Journal of Pharmacology*, **113**, 69–77.

CHAIMOWITZ, G. A., LINKS, P. S., PADGETT, R. W., et al (1991) Treatment-resistant depression: a survey of practice habits of Canadian psychiatrists. *Canadian Journal of Psychiatry*, **36**, 353–356.

COPPEN, A., SHAW, D. M. & FARRELL, J. P. (1963) Potentiation of the antidepressive effect of a monoamine-oxidase inhibitor by tryptophan. *Lancet*, **i**, 79–81.

COURNOYER, G., DE MONTIGNY, C., OVELLETTE, C., et al (1984) Lithium addition in tricyclic-resistant unipolar depression: a placebo-controlled study. Abstracts of 14th CINP Congress, Florence, F–177.

COWEN, P. J., McCANCE, S. L., COHEN, P. R., et al (1989) Lithium increases 5HT-mediated neuroendocrine responses in tricyclic resistant depression. *Psychopharmacology*, **99**, 230–232.

——, ——, WARE, C. J., et al (1991) Lithium in tricyclic-resistant depression: correlation of increased brain 5-HT function with clinical outcome. *British Journal of Psychiatry*, **159**, 341–346.

CULLEN, M., MITCHELL, P., BRODATY, H., et al (1991) Carbamazepine for treatment-resistant melancholia. *Journal of Clinical Psychiatry*, **52**, 472–476.

DALLAL, A., FONTAINE, R., ONTIVEROS, A., et al (1990) Lithium carbonate augmentation of desipramine in refractory depression. *Canadian Journal of Psychiatry*, **35**, 608–611.

DELGADO, P. L., PRICE, L. H., CHARNEY, D. S., et al (1988) Efficacy of fluvoxamine in treatment-refractory depression. *Journal of Affective Disorders*, **15**, 55–60.

DE MONTIGNY, C., GRUNBERG, F., MAYER, A., et al (1981) Lithium induces rapid relief of depression in tricyclic antidepressant drug non-responders. *British Journal of Psychiatry*, **138**, 252–256.

DINAN, T. G. & BARRY, S. (1989) A comparison of electroconvulsive therapy with a combined lithium and tricyclic combination among depressed tricyclic nonresponders. *Acta Psychiatrica Scandinavica*, **80**, 97–100.

DUGGAN, C. F., LEE, A. S. & MURRAY, R. M. (1990) Does personality predict long-term outcome in depression? *British Journal of Psychiatry*, **157**, 19–24.

EARLE, B. (1970) Thyroid hormone and tricyclic antidepressants in resistant depression. *American Journal of Psychiatry*, **126**, 1667–1669.

ECCLESTON, D., FERRIER, I. N. & MOORE, P. B. (1991) L-tryptophan and the treatment of chronic depression. Abstracts of Spring Quarterly Meeting, Royal College of Psychiatrists, p. 17.

FAWCETT, J., KRAVITZ, H. M., ZAJECKA, J. M., et al (1991) CNS stimulant potentiation of monoamine oxidase inhibitors in treatment-refractory depression. *Journal of Clinical Psychopharmacology*, **11**, 127–132.

FINK, M. (1989) Electroconvulsive therapy: the forgotten option in the treatment of therapy-resistant depression. *Treatment of Tricyclic-Resistant Depression* (ed. I. L. Extein), pp. 137–149. Washington, DC: American Psychiatric Press.

GARBUTT, J. C., MAYO, J. P., GILLETTE, G. M., et al (1986) Lithium potentiation of tricyclic antidepressants following lack of T_3 potentiation. *American Journal of Psychiatry*, **143**, 1038–1039.

GEORGOTAS, A., FRIEDMAN, E., McCARTHY, M., *et al* (1983) Resistant geriatric depressions and therapeutic response to monoamine oxidase inhibitors. *Biological Psychiatry*, **18**, 195–205.

——, McCUE, R. E., COOPER, T. B., *et al* (1989) Factors affecting the delay of antidepressant effect in responders to nortriptyline and phenelzine. *Psychiatry Research*, **28**, 1–9.

GEWIRTZ, G. R., MALASPINA, D., HATTERER, J. A., *et al* (1989) Occult thyroid dysfunction in patients with refractory depression. *American Journal of Psychiatry*, **145**, 1012–1014.

GLASSMAN, A. H., KANTOR, S. J. & SHOSTAK, M. (1975) Depression, delusions and drug response. *American Journal of Psychiatry*, **132**, 716–719.

GOODWIN, F. K., PRANGE, A. J. & POST, R. M. (1982) L-triiodothyronine converts tricyclic antidepressant non-responders to responders. *American Journal of Psychiatry*, **139**, 37–42.

GREENHOUSE, J. B., KUPFER, D. J., FRANK, E., *et al* (1987) Analysis of time to stabilisation in the treatment of depression: biological and clinical correlates. *Journal of Affective Disorders*, **13**, 259–266.

GUSCOTT, R. & GROF, P. (1991) The clinical meaning of refractory depression: a review for the clinician. *American Journal of Psychiatry*, **148**, 695–704.

HAMILTON, M. (1967) Development of a rating scale for primary depressive illness. *Journal of Social and Clinical Psychology*, **6**, 278–296.

HENINGER, G. R., CHARNEY, D. S. & STERNBERG, D. E. (1983) Lithium carbonate augmentation of antidepressant treatment – an effective prescription for treatment of refractory depression. *Archives of General Psychiatry*, **40**, 1335–1342.

JANICAK, P. G., DAVIS, J. M., GIBBONS, R. D., *et al* (1985) Efficacy of ECT – a meta-analysis. *American Journal of Psychiatry*, **142**, 297–302.

JOFFE, R. T., SINGER, W. & LEVITT, A. J. (1992) Methimazole in treatment-resistant depression. *Biological Psychiatry*, **31**, 1235–1237.

KANTOR, D., McNEVIN, S., LEICHNER, P., *et al* (1989) The benefit of lithium carbonate adjunct in refractory depression – fact or fiction. *Canadian Journal of Psychiatry*, **31**, 416–418.

KATONA, C. L. E. (1988) Lithium augmentation in refractory depression. *Psychiatric Developments*, **2**, 153–171.

KAY, D. S. G., NAYLOR, G. J., SMITH, A. H. W., *et al* (1984) The therapeutic effect of ascorbic acid and EDTA in manic–depressive psychosis: double blind comparisons with standard treatments. *Psychological Medicine*, **14**, 533–539.

KELLER, M. B., KLERMAN, G. L., LAVORI, P. W., *et al* (1982) Treatment received by depressed patients. *Journal of the American Medical Association*, **248**, 1848–1855.

——, ——, ——, *et al* (1984) Long-term outcome of episodes of major depression. *Journal of the American Medical Association*, **252**, 788–792.

—— & SHAPIRO, R. W. (1985) Double depression: superimposition of acute depressive episodes on chronic depressive disorders. *American Journal of Psychiatry*, **139**, 438–442.

LEONARD, B. E. (1988) Biochemical aspects of therapy-resistant depression. *British Journal of Psychiatry*, **152**, 453–459.

LEVITT, A. J., JOFFE, R. T. & KENNEDY, S. H. (1991) Bright light augmentation in antidepressant nonresponders. *Journal of Clinical Psychiatry*, **52**, 336–337.

MAGNI, G., FISMAN, M. & HELMES, E. (1988) Clinical correlates of ECT-resistant depression in the elderly. *Journal of Clinical Psychiatry*, **49**, 405–407.

McGRATH, P. J., STEWART, J. W., NUNES, E. V., *et al* (1993) A double-blind crossover trial of imipramine and phenelzine for outpatients with treatment-refractory depression. *American Journal of Psychiatry*, **150**, 118–123.

MURPHY, B. E., DHAR, V., GHADIRIAN, A. M., *et al* (1991) Response to steroid suppression in major depression resistant to antidepressant therapy. *Journal of Clinical Psychopharmacology*, **11**, 121–126.

MURPHY, E. (1983) The prognosis of depression in old age. *British Journal of Psychiatry*, **142**, 111–119.

NIERENBERG, A. A. (1991) Treatment choice after one antidepressant fails: a survey of northeastern psychiatrists. *Journal of Clinical Psychiatry*, **52**, 383–385.

―――― & AMSTERDAM, J. D. (1990) Treatment-resistant depression: definition and treatment approaches. *Journal of Clinical Psychiatry*, **51**(suppl. 6), 39–47.

―――― , PRICE, L. H., CHARNEY, D. S., *et al* (1990) After lithium augmentation: a retrospective follow-up of patients with antidepressant-refractory depression. *Journal of Affective Disorders*, **18**, 167–175.

NOLEN, W. A., VAN DE PUTTE, J. J., DIJKEN, W. A., *et al* (1988) Treatment strategy in depression II. MAO inhibitors in depression resistant to cyclic antidepressants: two controlled crossover studies with tranylcypromine versus L-5-hydroxytryptophan and nomifensine. *Acta Psychiatrica Scandinavica*, **78**, 676–683.

ONTIVEROS, A., FONTAINE, R. & ELIE, R. (1991) Refractory depression: the addition of lithium to fluoxetine or desipramine. *Acta Psychiatrica Scandinavica*, **83**, 188–192.

PARE, C. M. B. (1985) The present status of monoamine oxidase inhibitors. *British Journal of Psychiatry*, **146**, 576–584.

PRICE, L. H., CHARNEY, D. S. & HENINGER, G. R. (1985) Efficacy of lithium-tranylcypromine in refractory depression. *American Journal of Psychiatry*, **142**, 619–623.

―――― , ―――― & ―――― (1987) Reserpine augmentation of desipramine in refractory depression: clinical and neurobiological effects. *Psychopharmacology*, **92**, 431–437.

―――― , DELGADO, P. L., *et al* (1990) Fenfluramine augmentation in tricyclic-refractory depression. *Journal of Clinical Psychopharmacology*, **10**, 312–317.

RAZANI, J., WHITE, K., WHITE, J., *et al* (1983) The safety and efficacy of combined amitriptyline and tranylcypromine antidepressant treatment. *Archives of General Psychiatry*, **40**, 657–661.

REMICK, R. A. (1989) Treatment resistant depression. *Psychiatric Journal of the University of Ottawa*, **14**, 394–396.

ROOSE, S. P., GLASSMAN, A. H., WALSH, B. T., *et al* (1983) Depression, delusions and suicide. *American Journal of Psychiatry*, **140**, 1159–1162.

RYBAKOWSKI, J. & MATKOWSKI, K. (1992) Adding lithium to antidepressant therapy: factors related to therapeutic potentiation. *European Neuropsychopharmacology*, **2**, 161–165.

SCHMAUSS, M., LAAKMAN, G. & DIETERLE, D. (1988a) Effects of alpha-2 receptor blockade in addition to tricyclic antidepressants in therapy-resistant depression. *Journal of Clinical Psychopharmacology*, **8**, 108–111.

―――― , KAPFHAMMER, H. P., MEYR, P., *et al* (1988b) Combined MAO-inhibitor and tri-(tetra)cyclic antidepressant treatment in therapy resistant depression. *Progress in Neuropsychopharmacology and Biological Psychiatry*, **12**, 523–532.

SCHOPF, J., BAUMANN, P., LEMARCHAND, T., *et al* (1989) Treatment of endogenous depressions resistant to tricyclic antidepressants or related drugs by lithium addition. Results of a placebo-controlled double-blind study. *Pharmacopsychiatry*, **22**, 183–187.

SCHWEIZER, E., RICKELS, K., AMSTERDAM, J. D., *et al* (1990) What constitutes an adequate antidepressant trial for fluoxetine. *Journal of Clinical Psychiatry*, **51**, 8–11.

SETH, R., JENNINGS, A. L., BINDMAN, J., *et al* (1992) Combination treatment with noradrenalin and serotonin reuptake inhibitors in resistant depression. *British Journal of Psychiatry*, **161**, 562–565.

SHOPSIN, B. (1978) Enhancement of the antidepressant response to L-tryptophan by a liver pyrrolase inhibitor: a rational treatment approach. *Neuropsychobiology*, **4**, 188–192.

SIMPSON, G. M., LEE, J. H., CUCULIC, Z., *et al* (1976) Two dosages of imipramine in hospitalised endogenous and neurotic depressives. *Archives of General Psychiatry*, **33**, 1093–1102.

SPIKER, D. G., WEISS, J. C., DEALY, R. S., *et al* (1985) The pharmacological treatment of delusional depression. *American Journal of Psychiatry*, **142**, 430–436.

―――― , DEALY, R. S., HANN, I., *et al* (1986) Treating delusional depressives with amitriptyline. *Journal of Clinical Psychiatry*, **47**, 243–246.

STEIN, G. & BERNADT, M. (1993) Lithium augmentation therapy in tricyclic-resistant depression. A controlled trial using lithium in low and normal doses. *British Journal of Psychiatry*, **162**, 634–640.

THASE, M. E., KUPFER, D. J. & JARRETT, D. B. (1989a) Treatment of imipramine-resistant recurrent depression. I: an open clinical trial of adjunctive L-triiodothyronine. *Journal of Clinical Psychiatry*, **50**, 385–388.

——, ——, FRANK, E., *et al* (1989*b*) Treatment of imipramine-resistant recurrent depression. II: an open clinical trial of lithium augmentation. *Journal of Clinical Psychiatry*, **50**, 413–417.

——, FRANK, E., MALLINGER, A. G., *et al* (1992*a*) Treatment of imipramine-resistant recurrent depression. III: efficacy of monoamine oxidase-inhibitors. *Journal of Clinical Psychiatry*, **53**, 5–11.

——, MALLINGER, A. G., McKNIGHT, D., *et al* (1992*b*) Treatment of imipramine-resistant depression. IV: a double-blind crossover trial of tranylcypromine for anergic bipolar depression. *Americal Journal of Psychiatry*, **149**, 195–198.

WALINDER, J., SKOTT, A., CARLSSON, A., *et al* (1976) Potentiation of the antidepressant action of clomipramine by tryptophan. *Archives of General Psychiatry*, **33**, 1384–1389.

——, CARLSSON, A. & PERSSON, R. (1981) 5HT reuptake inhibitors plus tryptophan in endogenous depression. *Acta Psychiatrica Scandinavica*, **63**(suppl. 290), 179–190.

WEILBURG, J. B., ROSENBAUM, J. E., BIEDERMAN, J., *et al* (1989) Fluoxetine added to non-MAOI antidepressants converts nonresponders to responders: a preliminary report. *Journal of Clinical Psychiatry*, **50**, 447–449.

WHEATLEY, D. (1972) Potentiation of amitriptyline by thyroid hormone. *Archives of General Psychiatry*, **26**, 242–245.

WHITE, K., WYKOFF, W., TYNES, L.L., *et al* (1990) Fluvoxamine in the treatment of tricyclic-resistant depression. *Psychiatric Journal of the University of Ottawa*, **15**, 156–158.

WORRALL, E. P., MOODY, J. P., PEET, M., *et al* (1979) Controlled studies of the acute antidepressant effects of lithium. *British Journal of Psychiatry*, **135**, 255–262.

ZIMMER, B., ROSEN, J., THORNTON, J. E., *et al* (1991) Adjunctive lithium carbonate in nortriptyline-resistant elderly depressed patients. *Journal of Clinical Psychopharmacology*, **11**, 254–256.

ZUSKY, P. M., BIEDERMAN, J., ROSENBAUM, J. F., *et al* (1988) Adjunct low dose lithium carbonate in treatment-resistant depression: a placebo-controlled study. *Journal of Clinical Psychopharmacology*, **8**, 120–124.

8 Stereotactic subcaudate tractotomy in the management of severe psychiatric disorders

ANDREA L. MALIZIA

The psychosurgical operation of stereotactic subcaudate tractotomy is carried out in the UK for treatment-resistant depression, anxiety and obsessional disorders. Although only twenty such operations are carried out per year in the whole country, it is important that such a treatment option should remain available for these patients. This chapter discusses the operative procedure, indications, patient selection and characteristics, consent issues, side-effects, outcome and its possible predictors.

Brief history

The psychosurgical operation of stereotactic subcaudate tractotomy (SST) was developed in the 1960s by Knight (1965) who sought to refine the orbital undercut (Scoville, 1949), one of two modified ventro-medial operations commonly in use at the time for psychiatric illnesses, the other being bimedial leucotomy (Greenblatt & Solomon, 1952). Knight's aim was to achieve the same beneficial effects but to reduce side-effects. Observation led him to believe that the undercuts which had the greatest chance of success were those where the lesion extended below the head of the caudate nucleus. He then devised a method of lesioning the orbital subcaudate area selectively by the insertion of radioactive yttrium-90 rods under stereotactic control.

The effects of a more refined operation in terms of reduced postoperative morbidity and mortality have been striking. The immediate postoperative mortality is less than 1 in 1200, compared with 4% in standard leucotomy (Tooth & Newton, 1961) and 1.5% in orbital undercutting (Sykes & Tredgold, 1964). In fact, an operative error (Knight, 1973) precipitated the only death in the SST series in the UK since its inception. Postoperative epilepsy is about 2% (Goktepe et al, 1975) as compared with 10–15% in the cruder procedures. There seem to be no significant long-term neuropsychological effects (Bridges, 1972; Kartsounis et al 1991), and the impression is that illness factors have a far greater effect on the variance of the neuropsychological performance than the SST lesion. Patients do not develop the severe personality and volitional changes which occurred in the coarser procedures; although 7% of relatives report possible personality changes, these sometimes represent a return to normal function after years of inactivity (Goktepe *et al*, 1975). Some patients develop a postoperative acute confusional state; the proportion doing so has increased in recent years from less than 10% to about 25%, due to the fact that patients are not now requested to discontinue all their psychotropic medication before surgery.

Operative details

The operation has been fundamentally unchanged since its inception. Ten rods of yttrium-90, 7 mm in length and 1 mm in diameter and embedded in ceramic, are inserted bilaterally in two columns 1 mm apart and five rows 4 mm apart, with the help of a McCaul stereotactic frame and repeat air ventriculograms to calculate the siting empirically (Fig. 8.1). Patients do

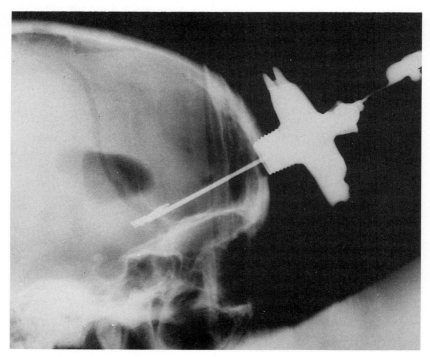

Fig. 8.1. Operative lateral air ventriculogram taken to check the position of the yttrium rods. The McCaul frame is still in position. At the end of the inserting cannula, the ceramic yttrium rods can be seen in place

not need to have their head shaved but do have a general anaesthetic. The incision is made in one of the skin creases in the forehead so as to be as cosmetically acceptable as possible, and two burr holes are made. The operation takes about 90 minutes, most of the time being spent taking air ventriculograms. Most patients are up and about within 24 hours of the surgery. There is considerable immediate postoperative oedema which is associated with a confusional state; this subsides, and at six months the lesion is circumscribed (Fig. 8.2) and entirely in the white matter of the orbital gyrus (Malizia *et al*, 1993).

About 20 SSTs are performed each year at the Brook Hospital, London, currently the only UK centre offering the treatment. These represent about 90% of the psychosurgical operations carried out in the UK every year. Since its inception, over 1200 tractotomies have been carried out in this unit. The team consists of a consultant neurosurgeon, a consultant psychiatrist, a ward doctor, an occupational therapist and a social worker. The team has at times been more restricted because of financial constraints, but the role of the two consultants working together is pivotal. While the neurosurgeon must retain the decision of whether to operate and can give definitive opinions about organic factors, the psychiatrist ensures that only patients with the

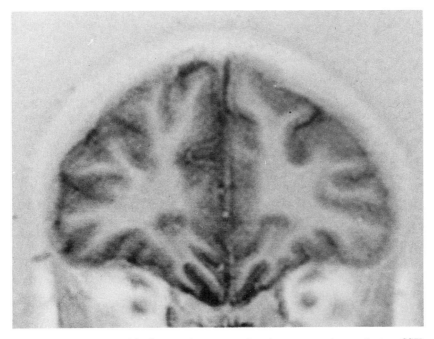

Fig. 8.2. A coronal T$_1$-weighted magnetic resonance imaging scan at six months post-SST, showing the lesion areas (dark) bilaterally in the white matter of the orbital gyrus

appropriate types of illness are operated on, and that all other appropriate treatments have been tried. Over the years this has resulted in more aggressive pharmacotherapeutic strategies being suggested by the psychiatrist (e.g. Hale *et al*, 1987); these have obviated the need for surgery in some patients.

Patient referral and consent

Most patients are referred by their local psychiatrist. For example, in a recent review of all the patients referred with bipolar affective disorder, two-thirds had been referred by the catchment area services and almost 20% were sent by other tertiary psychiatric centres. After assessment, and if the patients have already received adequate treatment, the procedure is explained. The patient's consent to the operation is not judged to be sufficient by English law, which requires a panel of one psychiatrist and two lay people appointed by the Mental Health Act commission to certify that the consent is 'free and full', as well as the psychiatrist (often not an expert in the procedure) certifying that it is an appropriate course of action. This has led to ethical debates when some patients have been too ill to comply with the mechanism as set in the law and have died (Bridges, 1992), or when patients refused surgery by the commission have committed suicide (Bridges, 1984, 1986).

Patient selection

Psychosurgery should be seen exclusively in the context of a treatment for affective, obsessional and anxiety disorders (Bartlett *et al*, 1981; Malizia & Bridges, 1991) that have not responded to all other reasonable forms of treatment. While in the early years patients with frank bipolar affective disorder were not selected, results in this disorder were found to be encouraging (Lovett & Shaw, 1987; Poynton *et al*, 1988) and by 1988–89 they represented 27% of referrals and 47% of operative procedures.

The purpose of the assessment procedure is, therefore, to establish that patients do have a severe psychiatric illness which is likely to respond, and that all other reasonable treatments have been attempted. Out of 100 referrals specifically for psychosurgery from 1988–89, 10% were inappropriate because patients had disorders not thought to respond to psychosurgery, and only about a quarter of patients with the appropriate diagnoses had reached a level of resistance which in our opinion warranted psychosurgery at the time of referral (Malizia & Bridges, 1992*b*). While it is felt that an adequate treatment algorithm is too rigid a structure to deal with the multiplicity of clinicians and patients, a recent review indicates the likely sequence of pharmacological manoeuvres which should be considered for treatment-resistant affective disorders (Malizia & Bridges, 1992*a*). For anxiety and obsessional disorders, evidence is also sought that appropriate cognitive–behavioural therapy has been carried out; availability of this sort of therapy is very variable throughout the country, and referral to a behaviour therapy specialist unit needs to be initiated.

Patient characteristics

A scrutiny of published and unpublished figures reveals that about 30% of SST patients are male (26% in Strom-Olsen & Carlisle (1971), and 33% between 1977 and 1992); for both sexes the average age at operation is in the early 50s. An average of 20 years had elapsed since the first episode of illness, with the current episode having lasted for an average of over five years. In one sample of patients with bipolar affective disorder, almost 70% were unable to sustain their usual work. These data indicate that patients who come for surgery are a very disabled group. It is often felt that earlier, more aggressive pharmacotherapy and continued prophylaxis along the lines set by the World Health Organization (WHO, 1989) could reduce this reservoir of despair.

Outcome

The beneficial effects of psychosurgery develop slowly over a period of three to ten months (Strom-Olsen & Carlisle, 1971). Hence outcome is assessed one year after surgery using a traditional five point scale (Pippard, 1955) used in many other psychosurgery studies. As well as a clinician's global rating, an estimate of social function is included (Bridges *et al*, 1973). The categories are:

    I. Recovered; no symptoms and no treatment required, full social function.
   II. Well; may be on treatment, mild or residual symptoms, little or no interference with daily life.
  III. Improved, but significant symptoms remain which interfere with the patient's life.
  IV. Unchanged.
   V. Worse.

Whenever this scale has been compared with more detailed standardised instruments such as the Present State Examination (Curson *et al*, 1983), the Wakefield Inventory or the Taylor Manifest Anxiety Scale (Goktepe *et al*, 1975), it has been shown to be robust, with fewer people being included in the good outcome categories than if just symptomatic improvement had been considered, because of the importance assigned to social functioning.

There has never been a controlled trial of this type of surgery; a protocol suggested at the inception of the Royal College of Psychiatrists (Barraclough, 1977) was never realised because of ethical and funding difficulties. At present two different strategies are being used as an attempt to use controls, one involving patients who were offered the surgery but did not agree to it, and one examining the effects of two periods in the last five years when long waiting lists developed because of technical problems with the manufacture of the rods. In addition, because the long-term effects of very high doses of antidepressant medication in combination are unknown, it may be considered ethical in the future to allocate patients randomly to either a 'superdose' treatment or surgery (Malizia & Bridges, 1993).

In this review, outcome results are collated from three early reviews (Strom-Olsen & Carlisle, 1971; Bridges *et al*, 1973; Goktepe *et al*, 1975) and from a recent personal audit of the results of SST between 1977 and 1992. The results are presented separately because of methodological differences; only the results for patients actually reassessed by the investigators are presented for the early studies, while this audit is based on a retrospective examination of the notes and has included outcome information supplied by referring psychiatrists or the patients themselves, but without the patient necessarily having been reassessed by the Unit's clinicians. In addition, diagnostic categories may not be entirely compatible between then and now. Results of this audit are comparable to another audit of the 1979–91 period (Hodgkiss *et al*, 1994).

Early studies

In total, 309 patients had a detailed reassessment. The results are presented in Table 8.1 and have been subdivided into diagnostic groups.

Recent audit

The recent audit was primarily concerned with an evaluation of patients with bipolar affective disorder (BP) who had the same twenty-rod lesion

TABLE 8.1
Early outcome studies

Diagnosis	Outcome					Total
	I	*II*	*III*	*IV*	*V*	
ON	22 (35%)	13 (11%)	15 (24%)	11 (19%)	1 (1%)	62
AS	21 (30%)	13 (19%)	16 (22%)	20 (29%)	0	70
Depression	64 (36%)	48 (27%)	39 (22%)	26 (15%)	0	177

ON = obsessional neurosis, AS = anxiety and tension states, depression = involutional, recurrent and other types.

between 1977 and 1992. For the purposes of comparison, outcome results for all the other patients operated on with the same lesion in the same period were also collected. In all, 66 patients with BP had been operated on, while 314 patients with other diagnoses also had SST. Reliable outcome information at one year follow-up was not available for three patients with BP and for 55 of the others. Results are presented in Table 8.2.

It can be seen that there has been a decline in the number of patients in the good outcome categories (I and II) since the early 1970s. While this conveys the initial impression that patients do not have as good an outcome, it poses the question of why this may be happening. The two major changes since the early 1970s have been that:

(a) a far lower proportion of operations is carried out for anxiety and obsessional disorders;
(b) the unit now insists that patients should have been tried on various treatment strategies before surgery (as set out in Malizia & Bridges, 1992*a*), while up to the mid-1970s all that was required was that antidepressants and ECT had been tried and that the referring consultant psychiatrist had tried all the treatment strategies that he or she felt were adequate.

Since the first of the two factors would have resulted in a slight improvement of the outcome figures, it is probable that the result of the more aggressive pharmacotherapeutic manoeuvres is that a more resistant population is now being selected for surgery than 20 years ago.

Suicide

Many studies have reported mortality by suicide of 8–15% (Guze & Robins, 1970; Kiloh *et al*, 1988) in groups of patients with severe affective disorders. In patients who have had SST the suicide rate is about 2–3%.

Measures predictive of outcome

Biological markers of depression (Malizia *et al*, 1990) and neuroendocrine measures (Corn *et al*, 1984) do not seem to be helpful in predicting the

TABLE 8.2
Audit of SST outcome in bipolar affective disorder, 1977–1992

Diagnosis	Outcome					Total
	I	*II*	*III*	*IV*	*V*	
BP	3 (5%)	23 (36%)	24 (38%)	12 (20%)	1 (1%)	63
Other	26 (10%)	67 (26%)	81 (31%)	79 (29%)	6 (4%)	259

BP = bipolar affective disorder, other = unipolar major depressive disorder, obsessive–compulsive disorder and panic disorder.

outcome from surgery. However, some biochemical (Pangalos *et al*, 1992), electrophysiological (Evans *et al*, 1981) and cerebral blood flow measures (Malizia *et al*, 1994) seem to correlate with outcome; unfortunately, none of these give preoperative predictors. Patients with cyclical and endogenomorphic features are preferentially selected, so that factor analyses of symptom profiles are not informative as they mirror selection biases. In an analysis of other factors affecting prognosis in patients with bipolar affective disorder, having a concomitant physical illness was associated with poorer outcome, while having a history of prominent anxiety or panic features and a definite family history of affective disorders were associated with a better outcome.

Conclusions

Almost 60 years have elapsed since the beginnings of modern psychosurgery. With the advent of psychotropics and an increased knowledge of their application, psychosurgery should only be considered in the treatment of affective, anxiety and obsessional disorders, and only when they do not respond to all other strategies. The older, coarser operations should be abandoned in favour of more selective ones such as SST or, for anxiety and obsessive–compulsive disorder, gamma-capsulotomy (Mindus, 1991) or stereotactic cingulotomy (Ballantine *et al*, 1987). There is often an emotional negative response to the word 'psychosurgery' which has dictated its demise in some countries. Psychiatrists in the UK have expressed, as a whole, a preference for such a treatment to continue to be available (Snaith *et al*, 1984), and ultimately referrers should remind themselves that consent lies with the patient. Until pharmacotherapeutic and other strategies can deal with all cases of intractable affective disorders, surgery should remain an option available to these profoundly disabled patients.

References

BALLANTINE, H. T., BOUCKOMS, A. J., THOMAS, E. I., *et al* (1987) Treatment of psychiatric illness by stereotactic cingulotomy. *Biological Psychiatry*, **22**, 807–819.

BARRACLOUGH, B. (1977) Evaluation of the surgical treatment of functional mental illness: proposal for a prospective controlled trial. In *Neurosurgical Treatment in Psychiatry, Pain and Epilepsy* (eds W. H. Sweet, S. Obrador & J. G. Martin-Rodriguez). Baltimore: Baltimore University Park Press.

BARTLETT, J. R., BRIDGES, P. K. & KELLY, D. (1981) Contemporary indications for psychosurgery. *British Journal of Psychiatry*, **38**, 507–511.

BRIDGES, P. K. (1972) Psychosurgery today: psychiatric aspects. *Proceedings of the Royal Society of Medicine*, 1104–1108 (Section of Psychiatry, 40–44).

——— (1984) Psychosurgery and the Mental Health Act Commission. *Psychiatric Bulletin*, **8**, 146–148.

——— (1986) The draft code of practice and psychosurgery (Correspondence). *Psychiatric Bulletin*, **10**, 212–213.

—— (1992) Is psychosurgery safer than Section 57? *Psychiatric Bulletin*, **16**, 510.

——, GOKTEPE, E. O. & MARATOS, J. (1973) A comparative review of patients with obsessional neurosis and with depression treated by psychosurgery. *British Journal of Psychiatry*, **123**, 663–674.

CORN, T. H., HONIG, A., THOMPSON, C., *et al* (1984) A neuroendocrine study of stereotactic subcaudate tractotomy. *British Journal of Psychiatry*, **144**, 417–420.

CURSON, D. A., TRAUER, T., BRIDGES, P. K., *et al* (1983) Assessment of outcome after psychosurgery using the Present State Examination. *British Journal of Psychiatry*, **143**, 118–123.

EVANS, B. M., BRIDGES, P. K. & BARTLETT, J. R. (1981) Electroencephalographic changes as prognostic indicators for psychosurgery. *Journal of Neurology, Neurosurgery and Psychiatry*, **44**, 444–447.

GOKTEPE, E. O., YOUNG, L. B. & BRIDGES, P. K. (1975) A further review of the results of stereotactic subcaudate tractotomy. *British Journal of Psychiatry*, **126**, 270–280.

GREENBLATT, M. & SOLOMON, H. C. (1952) Survey of nine years of lobotomy investigations. *American Journal of Psychiatry*, **109**, 262–265.

GUZE, S. B. & ROBINS, E. (1970) Suicide and primary affective disorders. *British Journal of Psychiatry*, **117**, 437–438.

HALE, A. S., PROCTER, A. & BRIDGES, P. K. (1987) Clomipramine, tryptophan and lithium in combination for resistant endogenous depression. Seven case studies. *British Journal of Psychiatry*, **151**, 213–217.

HODGKISS, A. D., MALIZIA, A. L., BARTLETT, J. R., *et al* (1994) Outcome after the psychosurgical operation of stereotactic subcaudate tractotomy 1979–1991. *Journal of Psychiatry and Clinical Neuroscience* (in press).

KARTSOUNIS, L., POYNTON, A. M., BARTLETT, J. R., *et al* (1991) Neuropsychological correlates of stereotactic subcaudate tractotomy; a prospective study. *Brain*, **114**, 2657–2673.

KILOH, L. G., ANDREWS, G. & NEILSON, M. (1988) The long term outcome of depressive illness. *British Journal of Psychiatry*, **153**, 752–757.

KNIGHT, G. (1965) Sterotactic tractotomy in the surgical treatment of mental illness. *Journal of Psychiatry*, **153**, 752–757.

—— (1973) Further observations from an experience of 660 cases of stereotactic tractotomy. *Postgraduate Medical Journal*, **49**, 845–854.

LOVETT, L. M. & SHAW, D. (1987) Outcome in bipolar affective disorder after stereotactic subcaudate tractotomy. *British Journal of Psychiatry*, **151**, 113–116.

MALIZIA, A. L., HALE, A. S., HANNAH, P., *et al* (1990) Tyramine sulphate excretion as a predictor of outcome in stereotactic subcaudate tractotomy. *Journal of Psychopharmacology*, **4**, 237.

—— & BRIDGES, P. K. (1991) Selecting patients for psychosurgery. In *Biological Psychiatry*, Vol. 2 (eds G. Racagni, N. Brunello & T. Fukada), pp. 224–226. Amsterdam: Excerpta Medica.

—— & —— (1992*a*) The management of treatment-resistant affective disorders: clinical perspectives. *Journal of Psychopharmacology*, **6**, 145–155.

—— & —— (1992*b*) A response to commentaries on treatment-resistant depression. *Journal of Psychopharmacology*, **6**, 172–175.

—— & —— (1993) The management of treatment-resistant affective disorder: a reply. *Journal of Psychopharmacology*, **7**, 91–95.

——, GRAVES, M. J., BINGHAM, J. B., *et al* (1993) Cerebral effects of stereotactic subcaudate tractotomy. In *Brain Imaging in Psychiatry* (ed. K. Maurer), pp. 57–60. Berlin: Springer-Verlag.

——, ALLEN, S., MAISEY, M., *et al* (1994) Changes in low frontal cerebral blood flow measured with Tc-99 HMPAO spect correlate with outcome in stereotactic subcaudate tractotomy carried out for treatment resistant depression. In *Refractory Depression* (eds J. Zohar, S. P. Roose & W. A. Nolen), pp. 163–167. Chichester: John Wiley.

MINDUS, P. (1991) *Capsulotomy in Anxiety Disorder: a Multidisciplinary Study*. Thesis. Stockholm: Karolinska Institute.

PANGALOS, M. N., MALIZIA, A. L., FRANCIS, P. T., *et al* (1992 Effect of psychotropic drugs on excitatory amino acids in patients undergoing psychosurgery for depression. *British Journal of Psychiatry*, **160**, 638–643.

PIPPARD, J. (1985) Rostral leucotomy; a report on 240 cases personally followed up after 1 to 5 years. *Journal of Mental Science*, **101**, 756–773.

POYNTON, A. M., BRIDGES, P. K. & BARTLETT, J. R. (1988) Resistant bipolar affective disorder treated by stereotactic subcaudate tractotomy. *British Journal of Psychiatry*, **152**, 354–358.

SCOVILLE, W. B. (1949) Selective cortical undercutting as means of modifying and studying frontal lobe function in man. *Journal of Neurosurgery*, **6**, 65–73.

STROM-OLSEN, R. & CARLISLE, S. (1971) Bifrontal stereotactic tractotomy. *British Journal of Psychiatry*, **118**, 141–154.

SYKES, M. K. & TREGOLD, R. F. (1964) Restricted orbital undercutting. A study of its effects on 350 patients over ten years, 1951–1960. *British Journal of Psychiatry*, **110**, 609–640.

TOOTH, G. C. & NEWTON, M. P. (1961) *Leucotomy in England and Wales, 1942–1954*. Ministry of Health Reports on Public Health and Medical Subjects, no. 104. London: HMSO.

WORLD HEALTH ORGANIZATION MENTAL HEALTH COLLABORATING CENTRES (1989) Pharmacotherapy of depressive disorders: a consensus statement. *Journal of Affective Disorders*, **17**, 197–198.

9 Obsessive–compulsive disorder – new pharmacological treatment directions

STUART A. MONTGOMERY, TIM BULLOCK, NAOMI FINEBERG and ANN ROBERTS

Obsessive–compulsive disorder (OCD) is a distressing and common condition. At one time it was thought to be a rather rare illness, with a prevalence of only around 0.5%. However, the early estimates of prevalence were biased by being based on hospitalised samples which did not represent the general population. There were, for example, no effective recognised treatments for severe forms of the disorder, and this would affect the recognition of OCD, the numbers and the type of patient admitted to hospital.

Recent epidemiological studies that have interviewed large random samples from the general population have shown that the prevalence of OCD is much higher than the early estimates suggest. The Epidemiological Catchment Area Study in the USA reported from a large (more than 18 000) sample that between 2.5 and 3% of the American public suffered from OCD with a level of severity that would satisfy the diagnostic criteria for OCD in DSM–III (American Psychiatric Association, 1980; Karno et al, 1988). Similar findings have been reported in other populations in Canada and New Zealand in studies that used the same methodology and assessment instruments. These studies employed lay raters to make the assessments and may well have underestimated the true prevalence, since even experienced clinicians frequently have difficulty in persuading some obsessional thinkers to reveal the extent of their ruminations.

Some criticism has been levelled at the higher prevalence estimates. It has been suggested that the DSM–III diagnostic criteria on which these estimates were based used a criterion of a minimum impairment of one hour's duration that is too mild. While it is true that many OCD sufferers spend most of their waking hours preoccupied with intrusive obsessional thoughts or rituals, preoccupation for at least one hour a day nevertheless represents a substantial intrusion into normal functioning. The percentage of the general population reporting this degree of impairment reveals the considerable level of morbidity associated with OCD in the community. This reduction in the ability to function underlines the need for effective treatment.

OCD is characterised by obsessions or compulsions (persistently recurring thoughts, impulses or urges) or rituals (repetitive behaviours that are apparently purposive but are neither preventative nor productive or are excessive). The thoughts or behaviours are not a source of pleasure, although they may reduce discomfort, and are time-consuming, distressing, and interfere with functioning. Obsessional thoughts or ruminations are regarded as the most common group, but it is clear that 90% of sufferers have mixed obsessions and compulsions (Rasmussen & Tsuang, 1986) with either obsessional thoughts or rituals being predominant.

The distinction between obsessional thoughts and rituals is not always evident since many obsessional thoughts have the quality of mental rituals. The separation is only relevant for treatment purposes because the ritualistic behaviours are the best targets for behavioural modification. The evidence from pharmacological studies shows that antiobsessional drugs are effective in improving both rituals and obsessional thoughts.

OCD and anxiety

There has been much discussion about the relationship of OCD to other psychiatric disorders. In Europe it has been customary to perceive OCD as a distinct diagnostic entity, and this view prevailed in the ICD–10 classification (World Health Organization, 1992) where obsessive–compulsive disorder maintains its separate status. Anxiety symptoms that frequently accompany the condition are regarded as secondary to or a part of the condition. This is at variance with the American approach which, in formulating the diagnostic system moved away from the distinctness of OCD embodied in DSM–II, and categorised OCD as an anxiety disorder in DSM–III and DSM–III–R (American Psychiatric Association, 1980, 1987). This approach does not appear to have been based on empirical evidence. There is indeed a growing body of evidence, drawn from clinical observation, biological studies and treatment studies, to suggest that OCD is a separate condition (Montgomery, 1992*b*).

There is no doubt that marked anxiety symptoms, both psychic and somatic, occur frequently in OCD, and approximately 6% of sufferers are also reported to have panic attacks (Rasmussen & Eisen, 1988). The occurrence of anxiety symptoms has tempted some observers to try to explain OCD in terms of anxiety symptoms, and this is reflected in DSM–III and the draft DSM–IV system. However, their occurrence is not of itself sufficient reason for categorising OCD as an anxiety disorder, and they are in any case not a prominent part of the presentation in all OCD patients. There are obvious differences between OCD and the anxiety disorders, including sex distribution, which is equal in OCD whereas the anxiety disorders occur in twice as many women as men, and the course of illness,

OCD being stable compared with anxiety disorders, which often develop into depression (Angst, 1990).

If OCD is an anxiety disorder, a therapeutic response to conventional anxiolytic drugs might be expected. Response to treatment alone cannot define a diagnostic category, but can provide a useful validation of diagnostic categories. Potential treatments that are considered to be anxiolytic are benzodiazepines, neuroleptics, and monoamine oxidase inhibitors. Some studies have been carried out to see if these drugs are effective in OCD, but the results have been disappointing (Trethowan & Scott, 1955; Rao, 1964; Orvin, 1967). Claims have been made for the efficacy of clonazepam on the basis of a crossover comparison of clomipramine and clonazepam with diphenhydramine as a control (Hewlett *et al*, 1992). Both clomipramine and clonazepam were reported to be effective compared with the control medication, but unfortunately the trial design, which did not include placebo and which may be affected by carryover effects of the multiple crossover, cannot adequately test efficacy.

Antidepressants with potent serotonin reuptake inhibition properties have provided the only successful pharmacotherapeutic intervention in OCD. The selective drugs of this class have been shown to have a differential advantage compared with conventional tricyclic antidepressants in treating the anxiety symptoms associated with depression (Montgomery, 1989, 1992*a*; Wakelin, 1988). This property does not, however, seem the likely mechanism by which they achieve their antiobsessional effect, given the lack of effect of conventional anxiolytics on either the anxiety or the obsessional symptoms.

OCD and depression

Many patients with OCD have depressive as well as obsessive/compulsive symptoms; a third may fulfil DSM–III–R criteria for major depression (Rasmussen & Eisen, 1992). These patients are likely to be diagnosed as having depression rather than OCD, partly because of difficulties in distinguishing between the ruminations of the depressed patient and obsessional ruminations. The DSM–III diagnostic criteria, which permitted the diagnosis of OCD only if depressive symptoms had not occurred earlier, may also have encouraged a preference for the diagnosis of depression. However, the importance of detecting OCD and making the diagnosis in spite of associated depressive symptoms has been demonstrated by the treatment studies.

OCD differs from depression in a number of important ways, including differences in the speed of response to effective drugs, the size and the course of response, and the response to placebo. The delay in response expected in depression is not characteristic of OCD. In three studies with clomipramine, response of OCD was seen as early as one to two weeks

(Montgomery, 1980; de Veaugh Geiss *et al*, 1989) but in major depression a significant difference from placebo cannot be reliably determined before four weeks. The response of OCD to placebo, with rates of 5% reported in the earlier studies, is lower than that seen in depression or in anxiety, which is routinely as high as 30%. The slow incremental improvement which continues over many weeks in OCD contrasts with major depression, which follows a more 'all or none' pattern of response during the acute episode followed by the need for continued consolidation treatment to prevent relapse.

The depressive symptoms seen in OCD follow a parallel response course of the obsessional symptoms, improving as the OCD improves, and this points to the two types of symptoms being part of the same process. They follow the same time-course of response as the obsessional symptoms and are not characterised by the delay which is usual in major depression. For example, in a placebo-controlled study of fluvoxamine (Goodman *et al*, 1989) the depressive symptoms showed the same early response as the obsessional symptoms and failed to show the substantial placebo response that would be expected in depression. The depressive symptoms are also seen to reappear on withdrawal of the drug as the obsessional symptoms deteriorate, as a discontinuation study of successful treatment with clomipramine showed (Pato *et al*, 1988).

Specificity of treatment

The most interesting aspect of pharmacotherapy in OCD is the selectivity of response to serotonergic agents. OCD does not respond to antidepressants without potent serotonergic effects even though these are effective in depression; nor do the depressive symptoms respond to all antidepressants, but only to those that are effective antiobsessional agents. It does not appear possible to treat the depressive symptoms in isolation; they have to be treated as integral to the OCD.

Conversely, antiobsessional drugs are effective in OCD in the presence or absence of depression, and it is therefore unlikely that the antiobsessional action is mediated by an antidepressant effect on the depressive symptoms, even though these are often profound. Initially it was thought that the efficacy of clomipramine, reported in an open study by Fernandez & Lopez Ibor (1967), was due to its known antidepressant effect. A direct test of whether the efficacy of clomipramine was specifically antiobsessional was made in 1980 by carrying out a placebo-controlled treatment study in patients for whom depression had been excluded (Montgomery, 1980). The demonstration of efficacy was later confirmed in another small study that excluded concomitant depression (Marks *et al*, 1988), and in two large multicentre studies (de Veaugh Geiss *et al*, 1989). Retrospective analyses of the results of studies that included patients with varying severities of depression have also reported that the initial severity of depressive symptoms did not appear to predict response.

Pharmacological treatment of OCD

The biological substrate of OCD is complex and poorly understood, but the evidence to suggest it is a disorder in which the serotonergic system plays a critical part in the evolution and treatment is impressive. The most telling evidence came initially from the clinical treatment studies.

The first effective pharmacological treatment for OCD, and for many years the most thoroughly investigated, was clomipramine. Its efficacy has been demonstrated with remarkable consistency. Five studies including patients with varying degrees of depression found clomipramine to be superior to placebo (Thoren *et al*, 1980; Marks *et al*, 1980; Insel *et al*, 1983, 1985; Flament *et al*, 1985; Mavissakalian *et al*, 1985) and four studies that excluded depression have shown that this effect was specifically antiobsessional (Montgomery, 1980; Marks *et al*, 1988; De Veaugh Geiss *et al*, 1989).

The clue that OCD might be a 'serotonin-specific' illness was provided by a lack of response to drugs that lacked potent serotoninergic action, which contrasted with the consistent efficacy of clomipramine. Neither of the selective noradrenaline reuptake inhibitors tested, nortriptyline and desipramine, were found to be effective, nortriptyline in a three-way study in which clomipramine was effective compared with placebo (Thoren *et al*, 1980), and desipramine in a small crossover study (Insel *et al*, 1985). The failure of desipramine was also seen in a direct comparison with clomipramine (Leonard *et al*, 1988). Amitriptyline and imipramine have been investigated, but without finding positive antiobsessional activity (Ananth *et al*, 1981; Foa *et al*, 1987) The failure of trazodone in a small placebo-controlled trial has also been interpreted as related to the weakness of its serotonergic actions (Piggott *et al*, 1992). The possibility that monoamine oxidase inhibitors may have an effect is still under review. Clorgyline was reported to be ineffective in an early study (Insel *et al*, 1983) but similar efficacy to clomipramine has been reported for phenelzine (Vallejo *et al*, 1992). This was, however, a small study without a placebo control, and caution is needed before ascribing efficacy to phenelzine.

Selective serotonin reuptake inhibitors

Clomipramine, although having potent effects in blocking serotonin reuptake, is not selective for serotonin and has a metabolite, desmethyl clomipramine, which is a potent noradrenaline reuptake inhibitor. The introduction of the class of antidepressants that are selective serotonin reuptake inhibitors (SSRIs) has made it possible to test further the relevance of serotonin for OCD. Additional treatments for OCD are needed because although clomipramine is an effective treatment and is widely used, it is a drug that is often associated with troublesome anticholinergic adverse events such as dry mouth, blurred vision and constipation. There is also a risk of seizure with clomipramine and a rate of 0.7% has been reported (Jermain & Crismon, 1990). The newer selective drugs are well tolerated and safer and therefore more suitable for patients with OCD, who worry about side-effects, and who are likely to be taking medication over prolonged periods.

Fluvoxamine was the earliest of the SSRIs to be investigated in OCD. There have now been five placebo-controlled studies, all of which have produced positive results. Three of the earlier studies were relatively small, being a crossover study of 20 patients (Perse *et al*, 1987), and two parallel group studies of 42 and 60 patients (Goodman *et al*, 1989; Cottraux *et al*, 1990). Subsequently, two large multicentre studies were carried out and these have confirmed that fluvoxamine is effective compared with placebo (Greist, 1991; Montgomery & Manceaux, 1992). As with clomipramine the efficacy of fluvoxamine did not depend on an antidepressant effect on depressive symptoms. Level of severity of depression at the start of the studies was not related to outcome (Goodman *et al*, 1989; Greist, 1991) and depressive symptoms improved with the obsessional symptoms (Perse *et al*, 1987; Price *et al*, 1987; Cottraux *et al*, 1990). Fluvoxamine was also compared to desipramine and, consistent with the findings with clomipramine, an antiobsessional effect was found for the SSRI but not with desipramine (Goodman *et al*, 1990).

Antiobsessional efficacy appears to be a class effect of the SSRIs since all those that have been tested have been found to be effective. Sertraline, for example, was found to be effective compared with placebo in two large multicentre studies, one of which compared different dosages (Chouinard *et al*, 1990; Chouinard, 1992). Two placebo-controlled multicentre studies have shown the efficacy of fluoxetine (Wheadon, 1991; Montgomery & Manceaux, 1992).

Therapeutic doses

Many experienced clinicians believe that higher doses of antiobsessional drugs are associated with greater efficacy in OCD. Higher doses often carry a greater side-effects burden and this can be a problem with a drug with a high level of side-effects such as clomipramine. The optimum dose of clomipramine has not been properly established in direct comparisons of different dose levels, although there is evidence that lower doses of 75 mg and 150 mg have efficacy (Montgomery, 1980; Thoren *et al*, 1980).

Doses of 50, 100 and 200 mg of sertraline have been directly compared, and there was no significant differences in response between them, suggesting that any advantage of higher doses may be small. However, the response effect was greatest at the 200 mg dose. There are contradictory results with fluoxetine. In the multicentre study carried out in Europe, best evidence of efficacy was seen with the 60 mg dose, the 40 mg dose was also effective, but the evidence for the 20 mg dose of fluoxetine was equivocal (Montgomery *et al*, 1993). In the larger study carried out in the USA, all three doses of fluoxetine were effective with little difference between them (Wheadon, 1991). The results with fluoxetine suggest that low doses are effective, but as better efficacy was seen with high doses in one study it is possible that there may be a subgroup of patients in whom high doses are needed. For those who do need higher doses of antiobsessional drugs, the safety profile of the drug becomes very important.

Refractory OCD

A substantial number of patients suffering from OCD show a poor response to treatment with SSRIs, and alternative strategies are still needed. One suggested approach to management of the refractory patient is to add a drug with serotonergic action to an SSRI. Adjunctive therapy with lithium has been shown to be effective in improving response to antidepressants (including SSRIs) in depression, but this approach has not been successful in OCD. This may be because lithium's serotonergic activity does not occur in the brain regions thought to be most closely involved in OCD (Blier & de Montigny, 1992). Adding buspirone to SSRIs to try to increase the effect at the 5-HT_{1A} receptor also appears unsuccessful (McDougle *et al*, 1990; Grady *et al*, 1993).

The only adjunctive treatment with good evidence of extra efficacy is neuroleptics added to SSRIs (McDougle *et al*, 1990). In examining the possible causes of non-response, the evidence suggesting a role for dopamine in the pathophysiology of OCD or in subgroups of OCD was noted. The marked association between OCD and a number of disorders in which basal ganglia dysfunction plays an important role, added to the indications of basal ganglia involvement in OCD as seen in PET scanning studies, suggests a possible neurological basis (von Economo, 1931; Baxter *et al*, 1987, 1988; Swedo *et al*, 1989). The exploration of the neuropathology that may underlie OCD is still at a very early stage, however, and the mechanisms between any reported cerebral changes and the illness have still to be determined. Dopamine antagonists alone are ineffective in treating OCD, but in the study of refractory OCD carried out by McDougle *et al* (1990) the addition of low-dose dopamine antagonists to ongoing SSRI therapy produced an improvement in those patients who had associated tics. The combination treatment was not effective in patients without tics. The authors suggest that where OCD is associated with chronic tics, this combination may be more effective than the SSRI alone.

Long-term treatment

OCD usually has a chronic fluctuating course, although episodic cases are recognised (Ravizza *et al*, 1993). Response is not usually rapid, with step-by-step improvement by small increments which may not be fully apparent until three months or later. Treatment is likely to be a long-term phenomenon measured in months or years rather than weeks. Long-term outcome has not been thoroughly studied and we do not have clear answers to the question of whether pharmacological treatment is effective over the long-term, and how long should it be continued.

There are reports in the literature that selected groups of responders remained improved for up to one year, but the lack of a placebo control compromises these reports. Some information is gained from the double-blind extension treatment given to responders in acute treatment studies with clomipramine, with sertraline, and with fluoxetine, and the response obtained on the drugs appears to be maintained over the one-year periods examined (Katz *et al*, 1990; Greist *et al*, 1992; Montgomery *et al*, 1993). Adequate direct tests of long-term efficacy using a randomised placebo-controlled discontinuation design are generally lacking. However, the study reported by Pato *et al* (1988) indicated the need for long-term treatment with clomipramine in view of the rapid worsening of obsessive–compulsive symptomatology when placebo was substituted double-blind for clomipramine.

Conclusions

The response in OCD is mostly partial and patients are left with some residual symptoms. This seems disappointing, but the partial symptomatic response is associated with substantial improvement in social and occupational function, as preoccupation with obsessions or rituals is reduced. It is a common experience that a rating scale of OCD symptoms will show only little change in a patient who has responded, whereas a global scale of improvement shows marked amelioration.

The advent of the SSRIs has been welcomed as an effective and well tolerated treatment for OCD. It is, however, the experience of many clinicians that the best response is when treatment with antiobsessional drugs and behaviour therapy are combined. There is no evidence that drugs and behavioural treatments interfere with each other. The evidence for efficacy of drug therapy is strongest in the patients with more severe symptoms rather than milder symptoms, when behaviour therapy appears most helpful. A strategy for management would be to initiate treatment with antiobsessional drugs, and to introduce behavioural treatments when partial response begins to be seen and patients are better able to benefit from a behavioural regime.

References

AMERICAN PSYCHIATRIC ASSOCIATION (1980) *Diagnostic and Statistical Manual of Mental Disorders* (3rd edn) (DSM–III). Washington, DC: APA.
────── (1987) *Diagnostic and Statistical Manual of Mental Disorders* (3rd edn, revised) (DSM–III–R). Washington, DC: APA.
ANANTH, J., PECKNOLD, J. C., VAN DEN STEEN, N., *et al* (1981) Double-blind comparative study of clomipramine and amitriptyline in obsessive neurosis. *Progress in Neuropsychopharmacology and Biological Psychiatry*, **5**, 257–262.
ANGST, J. (1990) Natural history and epidemiology of depression. In *Current Approaches* (eds J. Cobb & N. Goeting) pp. 1–11. Southampton: Duphar Medical Relations.
BAXTER, L. R., PHELPS, M. E., MAZZIOTTA, J. C., *et al* (1987) Local cerebral glucose metabolic rates in obsessive–compulsive disorder. A comparison with rates in unipolar depression and in normal controls. *Archives of General Psychiatry*, **44**, 211–218.
──────, SCHWARTZ, J. M., MAZZIOTTA, J. C., *et al* (1988) Cerebral glucose metabolic rates in non-depressed obsessive–compulsives. *American Journal of Psychiatry*, **145**, 1560–1563.
BLIER, P. & DE MONTIGNY, C. (1992) Lack of efficacy of lithium augmentation in obsessive–compulsive disorder: the perspective of different regional effects of lithium on serotonin release in the central nervous system. *Journal of Clinical Psychopharmacology*, **12**, 65–66.
CHOUINARD, G. (1992) Sertraline in the treatment of obsessive compulsive disorders: two double-blind, placebo controlled studies. *International Clinical Psychopharmacology*, **7**, 37–41.
──────, GOODMAN, W., GREIST, J., *et al* (1990) Results of a double blind serotonin uptake inhibitor sertraline in the treatment of obsessive compulsive disorder. *Psychopharmacology Bulletin*, **26**, 279–284.
COTTRAUX, J., MOLLARD, E., BOUVARD, M., *et al* (1990) A controlled study of fluvoxamine and exposure in obsessive compulsive disorders. *International Clinical Psychopharmacology*, **5**, 17–30.
DE VEAUGH GEISS, J., LANDAU, P. & KATZ, R. (1989) Treatment of obsessive compulsive disorder with clomipramine. *Psychiatry Annals*, **19**, 97–101.
FERNANDEZ, C. E. & LOPEZ-IBOR, J. J. (1967) Monochlorimipramine in the treatment of psychiatric patients resistant to other therapies. *Actas Luso-Espanolas de Neurologia, Psiquiatria y Ciensias Afine*, **26**, 119–147.
FLAMENT, M., RAPOPORT, J. & BERG, C. (1985) Clomipramine treatment of childhood OCD: a double-blind controlled study. *Archives of General Psychiatry*, **42**, 977–983.
FOA, E., STEKETEE, G., KOZAK, M., *et al* (1987) Imipramine and placebo in the treatment of obsessive compulsives: their effect on depression and obsessional symptoms. *Psychopharmacology Bulletin*, **23**, 8–11.
GOODMAN, W. K., PRICE, L. H., RASMUSSEN, S. A., *et al* (1989) Efficacy of fluvoxamine in obsessive compulsive disorder. *Archives of General Psychiatry*, **46**, 36–44.
──────, ──────, DELGADO, P. L., *et al* (1990) Specificity of serotonin reuptake inhibitors in the treatment of obsessive compulsive disorder. *Archives of General Psychiatry*, **47**, 577–585.
GRADY, T. A., PICOTT, T. A., L'HEUREUX, F., *et al* (1993) Double-blind study of adjuvant buspirone for fluoxetine-treated patients with obsessive–compulsive disorder. *American Journal of Psychiatry*, **150**, 819–821.
GREIST, J. H. (1991) Fluvoxamine treatment of obsessive-compulsive disorder. Presented at 5th World Congress of Biological Psychiatry, Florence.
──────, CHOUINARD, G., DUBOFF, E., *et al* (1992) Long-term sertraline treatment of obsessive compulsive disorder: a 52-week double-blind comparative study versus placebo. Presented at 31st Annual Meeting of the American College of Neuropsychopharmacology, Puerto Rico.

HEWLETT, W. A., VINOGRADOV, S. & AGRAS, W. S. (1992) Clomipramine, clonazepam, and clonidine treatment of obsessive compulsive disorder. *Journal of Clinical Psychopharmacology*, **12**, 420–430.

INSEL, R. R., MUELLER, E. A., ALTERMAN, I., *et al* (1985) Obsessive compulsive disorder and serotonin: is there a connection? *Biological Psychiatry*, **20**, 1174–1188.

——, MURPHY, D. L., COHEN, R. M., *et al* (1983) Obsessive compulsive disorder – a double blind trial of clomipramine and clorgyline. *Archives of General Psychiatry*, **40**, 605–612.

JERMAIN, D. M. & CRISMON, M. L. (1990) Pharmacotherapy of obsessive compulsive disorder. *Pharmacotherapy*, **10**, 175–198.

KARNO, M., GOLDING, J., SORENSON, S., *et al* (1988) The epidemiology of obsessive compulsive disorder in five US communities. *Archives of General Psychiatry*, **49**, 1094–1099.

KATZ, R. J., DE VEAUGH GEISS, J. & LANDAU, P. (1990) Clomipramine in obsessive compulsive disorder. *Biological Psychiatry*, **28**, 401–414.

LEONARD, H., SWEDO, S., RAPOPORT, J., *et al* (1988) Treatment of childhood obsessive compulsive disorder with clomipramine and desmethylimipramine: a double blind crossover comparison. *Psychopharmacology Bulletin*, **24**, 93–95.

MARKS, I. M., LELLIOTT, P., BASOGLU, M., *et al* (1988) Clomipramine, self exposure and therapist aided exposure for obsessive compulsive rituals. *British Journal of Psychiatry*, **152**, 522–534.

——, STERN, R. S., MAWSON, D., *et al* (1980) Clomipramine and exposure for obsessive compulsive rituals. *British Journal of Psychiatry*, **136**, 1–25.

MAVISSAKALIAN, M., TURNER, S., MICHELSON, L., *et al* (1985) Tricyclic antidepressants in obsessive disorder: antiobsessional or antidepressant agents. *American Journal of Psychiatry*, **142**, 572–576.

MCDOUGLE, C. J., PRICE, L. H., GOODMAN, W. K., *et al* (1990) Neuroleptic addition in fluvoxamine – refractory obsessive–compulsive disorder. *American Journal of Psychiatry*, **147**, 652–654.

——, GOODMAN, W. K., PRICE, L. H., *et al* (1991) Neuroleptic addition in fluvoxamine-refractory obsessive–compulsive disorder. *American Journal of Psychiatry*, **147**, 652–654.

MONTGOMERY, S. A. (1980) Clomipramine in obsessional neurosis: a placebo controlled trial. *Pharmaceutical Medicine*, **1**, 189–192.

—— (1989) The efficacy of fluoxetine as an antidepressant in the short and long term. *International Clinical Psychopharmacology*, **4** (suppl. 1), 113–119.

—— (1992*a*) The advantages of paroxetine in different subgroups of depression. *International Clinical Psychopharmacology*, **6** (suppl. 4), 91–100.

—— (1992*b*) OCD floats free of anxiety. *European Neuropsychopharmacology*, **2** (suppl. 2), 217–218.

—— & MANCEAUX, A. (1992) Fluvoxamine in the treatment of obsessive compulsive disorder. *International Clinical Psychopharmacology*, **7** (suppl. 1), 5–9.

——, MCINTYRE, A., OSTERHEIDER, M., *et al* (1993) A double-blind placebo-controlled study of fluoxetine in patients with DSM–III–R obsessive–compulsive disorder. *European Neuropsychopharmacology*, **3**, 143–152.

ORVIN, G. H. (1967) Treatment of the phobic obsessive compulsive patient with oxazepam: an improved benzodiazepine compound. *Psychosomatics*, **8**, 278–280.

PATO, M., ZOHAR-KADOUCH, R., ZOHAR, J., *et al* (1988) Return of symptoms after discontinuation of clomipramine in patients with obsessive compulsive disorder. *American Journal of Psychiatry*, **145**, 1543–1548.

PERSE, T. L., GREIST, J. H., JEFFERSON, J. W., *et al* (1987) Fluvoxamine treatment of obsessive compulsive disorder. *American Journal of Psychiatry*, **144**, 1543–1548.

PIGGOTT, T. A., L'HEUREUX, F., RUBENSTEIN, C. S., *et al* (1992) A double-blind placebo-controlled study of trazodone in patients with obsessive-compulsive disorder. *Journal of Clinical Psychopharmacology*, **12**, 156–162.

PRICE, L. H., GOODMAN, W. K., CHARNEY, D. S., *et al* (1987) Treatment of severe obsessive-compulsive disorder with fluvoxamine. *American Journal of Psychiatry*, **144**, 1059–1061.

RAO, A. V. (1964) A controlled trial with "Valium" in obsessive–compulsive states. *Journal of Indian Medical Association*, **42**, 564–567.

RASMUSSEN, S. A. & TSUANG, M. T. (1986) Clinical characteristics and family history in DSM–III obsessive compulsive disorder. *American Journal of Psychiatry*, **143**, 317–322.

―――― & EISEN, J. L. (1988) Clinical and epidemiologic findings of significance to neuropharmacologic trials in OCD. *Psychopharmacology Bulletin*, **24**, 466–470.

―――― & EISEN, J. L. (1992) Epidemiology of obsessive compulsive disorder. *Journal of Clinical Psychiatry*, **51**, 10–15.

RAVIZZA, L., MAINA, G., ROCCA, P., *et al* (1993) Biological and therapeutic aspects of obsessive compulsive disorder. Presented at 1st International OCD Conference, Capri.

SWEDO, S. E., RAPOPORT, J. L., CHESLOW, D. L., *et al* (1989) High prevalence of obsessive–compulsive symptoms in patients with Sydenham's chorea. *American Journal of Psychiatry*, **146**, 246–249.

THOREN, P., ASBERG, M., CRONHOLM, B., *et al* (1980) Clomipramine treatment in obsessive compulsive disorder. I: A controlled clinical trial. *Archives of General Psychiatry*, **37**, 1281–1285.

TRETHOWAN, W. H. & SCOTT, P. A. L. (1955) Chlorpromazine in obsessive–compulsive and allied disorders. *Lancet*, **1**, 781–785.

VALLEJO, J., OLIVARES, J., MARCOS, T., *et al* (1992) Clomipramine versus phenelzine in obsessive compulsive disorder. A controlled clinical trial. *British Journal of Psychiatry*, **161**, 665–670.

VON ECONOMO, C. (1931) *Encephalitis Lethargica: its Sequelae and Treatment*. Oxford: Oxford University Press.

WAKELIN, J. (1988) The role of serotonin in depression and suicide: do serotonin reuptake inhibitors provide a key? *Advances in Biological Psychiatry*, **17**, 70–83.

WHEADON, D. (1991) A placebo-controlled multicentre trial of fluoxetine in OCD. Presented at 5th World Congress of Biological Psychiatry, Florence.

Part IV. Psychological interventions

10 Cognitive–behavioural approaches to obsessive–compulsive disorder

JEAN COTTRAUX and DANIEL GÉRARD

In the last 15 years a behavioural method, exposure and response prevention, has demonstrated its effectiveness in obsessive–compulsive disorder (OCD) management (Marks, 1987). Meanwhile, evidence has appeared in favour of a specific effect of serotonergic antidepressants on rituals. Four drugs have been tested or retested in recent controlled trials: clomipramine (The Clomipramine Collaborative Group, 1991), fluvoxamine (Goodman *et al*, 1989), fluoxetine (Montgomery, 1992) and sertraline (Greist *et al*, 1992). Their effects on rituals and obsessive thoughts are independent of the level of depression. However, their use raises some problems; relapses are common after drug withdrawal, and side-effects, especially anorgasmia, are a frequent problem during clomipramine treatment (Monteiro *et al*, 1986). Therefore, the advantages of psychological treatments should be compared with those of medication and their combination.

Antidepressants and exposure

Clomipramine

Solyom & Sookman (1977), in a controlled study ($n = 27$), compared clomipramine with exposure (*in vivo* and in the imagination) and thought stopping. After six months clomipramine was as effective as exposure, but more effective than thought stopping in reducing ruminations. Clomipramine was less effective than exposure in reducing rituals. This suggests that the combination of the two treatments might be useful when rituals and ruminations occur together.

One study (Marks *et al*, 1980; Stern *et al*, 1980) found a short-term effect of clomipramine on rituals, mood and social adjustment in 40 moderately depressed OCD patients (mean Hamilton depression score = 18), but only in patients with initial depressed mood. At two-year follow-up there was no drug effect but a stable exposure effect. Another study (Marks *et al*, 1988) with 49 non-depressed OCD patients (mean Hamilton depression score = 8) found that clomipramine played a limited adjuvant short-term role, and therapist-guided exposure a marginal one. The most important factor was self-exposure at the end of treatment and at two- and six-year follow-ups. These two latter controlled studies suggested that clomipramine was useful only in depressed OCD patients, while exposure was sufficient for non-depressed patients.

Fluvoxamine

Cottraux *et al* (1990) randomly assigned 60 OCD patients (mean Hamilton depression scale = 19) to fluvoxamine with anti-exposure, fluvoxamine with exposure, or placebo with exposure for 24 weeks. All three groups improved in rituals and depression. At week 8 there was a between-group drug effect on rituals, but not on depression. At week 24 there was a between-group drug effect on depression, but not on rituals. At week 48 there was no between-group difference in rituals or depression. Discriminant analysis searching for posterior prediction of success or failure at post-test showed that higher avoidance scores predicted 68% of the correctly classified patients in the whole sample. No between-group difference was found in the predictive power of the discriminant function (Cottraux *et al*, 1993).

At a 12-month post-treatment follow-up (Cottraux *et al*, 1993), patients ($n = 33$) on the whole remained improved with no between-group differences. Over 80% of the fluvoxamine with exposure and placebo with exposure patients, versus 40% of fluvoxamine with anti-exposure patients, were not on antidepressants ($P < 0.05$). In summary, fluvoxamine and exposure were synergistic in the short term, and exposure reduced subsequent antidepressants in the follow-up year after both treatments had been stopped.

Imipramine

Foa *et al* (1992) divided 38 OCD patients into depressed and non-depressed subsamples on the basis of their depression (mean Hamilton depression score 20 or 11). Subjects in each subsample were randomly assigned to either imipramine or placebo for a period of 22 weeks. Medication was administered alone for the first six weeks. Then both groups received three weeks of intensive *in vitro* and *in vivo* exposure with response prevention, followed by 12 weekly sessions of supportive therapy. The post-treatment follow-up was of two years. Six weeks of imipramine alone reduced depression among depressed patients but did not modify obsessions or compulsions, which were improved only when exposure was added. Improvement in obsessive–compulsive symptoms was comparable in both placebo plus exposure and imipramine plus exposure groups, suggesting it was due to exposure.

Fluoxetine

Baxter *et al* (1992) compared nine patients treated with exposure, associated with group cognitive intervention, with nine patients treated with fluoxetine. Both groups were treated for ten weeks. Patients were not depressed (mean Hamilton depression score = 9). Both groups improved with no difference at post-test. Moreover, baseline hypermetabolism, assessed with an [18]fluorodeoxyglucose positron emission tomography (PET) scan of the right caudate nucleus, was decreased in patients who responded to either fluoxetine or exposure. The study suggested that the right caudate hypermetabolism was a state marker. The response was broader with fluoxetine, which also produced a metabolic decrease in the right cingulum and left thalamus.

Cognitive therapy (CT) and exposure

Limitations of exposure treatments (refusal, relapses and resistance in carrying out exposure homework) led to the design of new therapies to modify enduring cognitive processes and structures. Emmelkamp *et al* (1980) did not find that adding self-instructional training (SIT) to *in vivo* exposure gave a superior effect. SIT encourages patients (*n* = 15) to modify self-statements and replace negative thoughts with positive ones. Failure of SIT can be explained by the fact that it could have been used by the patients as a cognitive ritual, fighting the obsessive idea. Later, Emmelkamp *et al* (1988) compared cognitive therapy (CT: modification of obsessive thoughts and basic schemata) without exposure, with exposure *in vivo* in mild OCD (*n* = 18). Six months after the end of the treatment, both groups showed equivalent reductions in rituals, generalised anxiety, and social anxiety, but only the group receiving CT presented a positive change on depression measures. In a more impaired sample (*n* = 21), Emmelkamp & Beens (1991) found that CT and *in vivo* exposure had been equally effective at a six-month post-treatment follow-up. Nevertheless, larger studies are needed to establish the effectiveness of 'pure' CT in OCD.

Guidelines for clinical management

For non-depressed OCD patients, exposure is the treatment of choice. It has no side-effects, is long-lasting and does not create dependence. Non-depressed OCD patients who refuse exposure could receive, on a long-term basis, high doses of serotonergic antidepressant treatment instead (e.g. 225 mg of clomipramine, 300 mg of fluvoxamine, 40–80 mg of fluoxetine, or 50–200 mg of sertraline). Combined treatment is recommended in depressed OCD, the effects of combination being broader and more rapid than those of exposure alone, and the combination allowing drug cessation more frequently than medication alone.

Future research should address three main issues: (a) a large-scale study comparing six months of exposure with medication, alone or combined, over three years is now overdue; (b) the optimal length of serotonergic antidepressant treatment has to be defined; (c) the effects of cognitive therapy on both depression and rituals in OCD have to be tested further and compared with those of antidepressants.

Towards an information processing model

Cognitive model

A cognitive model of OCD has been proposed by Salkovskis (1985). Intrusive repugnant or antisocial thoughts, provoked by external or internal stimuli, activate automatic guilt and responsibility schemata. Negative appraisal of intrusive thoughts by these schemata results in neutralisations which are intentional, covert or overt responses intending to reduce abnormal guilt and responsibility feelings. Hence, habituation of intrusive thoughts does not occur. Intrusive thoughts are found in more than 80% of normal subjects (Rachman & Da Silva, 1978; Salkovskis & Harrison, 1984; Freeston *et al*, 1991). Abnormal and normal intrusive thoughts do not differ in content, but in rejectability, duration, frequency and habituation.

Neuropsychological and psychometric studies

Sauteraud *et al* (1992) compared 24 non-depressed OCD patients with 21 normal subjects on three lexical decision experiments using neutral, obsessive and guilt target words. OCD patients did not differ from control subjects in processing neutral words and guilt words, but they were significantly slower than controls when processing obsessive target words. The delay spread to pseudo-words when presented in the same experiment as obsessive words. These outcomes are compatible with Salkovskis' (1985) model, but the relation of intrusion to possible guilt schemata remains to be demonstrated, as shown by Ilai *et al* (1991) in a Stroop test experiment. Moreover, using the Perceived Guilt Index in a normal population, Reynolds & Salkovskis (1991) failed to replicate a predictive relation between guilt and intrusive thoughts or impulses found in another study (Niler & Beck, 1989).

Neuroimagery studies

PET and single photon emission computerised tomography (SPECT) technology has been used to analyse intrusive thoughts or images while processed by the brain. Zohar *et al* (1989) studied cerebral blood flow with SPECT in ten OCD patients under three conditions: imaginal flooding, relaxation, and *in vivo* exposure. Cerebral blood flow decreased during *in vivo* exposure in parieto-occipital regions, but was increased in the temporal region during imaginal flooding. It was suggested that habituation was linked to brain stem activity, and accompanied by a decrease of higher order functions. Repeated *in vivo* exposure could be associated with increased cerebral blood flow, reflecting the re-establishment of higher order functions with greater degrees of cognitive processing as a result of 'reality testing'.

Several PET and SPECT studies strongly suggest that OCD patients show hypermetabolism in the caudate nuclei and/or frontal lobes, the most common finding being hyperfrontality (Baxter *et al*, 1987, 1988, 1992; Nordhal *et al*, 1989; Swedo *et al*, 1989; Benkelfat *et al*, 1990; Sawle *et al*, 1991; Machlin *et al*, 1991).

Baxter *et al* (1992) proposed a tentative model. The caudate nucleus could be a mediator between the orbito-frontal cortex, the thalamus and obsessive–compulsive behaviours. Obsessive impulses and thoughts are processed by the striatum, the left fronto-orbital cortex and the cingulate gyri. The striatum may suppress adventitious thoughts, sensations and actions without intervention of any cortical management. An inadequate filtering or suppression of frontal worry inputs may explain the struggle between intrusive thoughts and neutralising thoughts or motor rituals. The hypermetabolism found in the caudate nucleus and frontal orbital gyrus may reflect the obsessive struggle.

However, other authors, also comparing OCD with controls, reported a hypometabolism in orbital gyri and caudate nuclei (Mindus *et al*, 1989) or in the whole cortex (Martinot *et al*, 1990). In the Mindus *et al* (1989) study, which included patients before psychosurgery, this might be related to the long duration of the illness, with a final breakdown of resistance to obsessive thoughts and rituals. The effects of drugs cannot be ruled out in the Martinot *et al* (1990) study; ten of the 16 patients were under medication. Across-centre differences in PET technology or delineation of the regions of interest may also account for discrepant findings. Moreover, the patient's emotions and cognitions may modify local metabolism or cerebral blood flow. A ^{15}O-PET-scan study (Cottraux *et al*, 1992) is now nearing completion, comparing rest, neutral and obsessive auditory stimulations in unmedicated OCD patients with checking rituals versus controls.

Conclusions

Studies on information processing in OCD seem a promising new frontier, associating behavioural, cognitive and biological research. Further studies are needed to test the different levels of the model: biology of habituation process; psychophysiology of suppression; psychological effects of intrusive thoughts; relation of intrusions to possible guilt-responsibility schemata, and their development from early experiences. This model should also account for the therapeutic effects of exposure, cognitive therapy and serotonergic antidepressants.

References

BAXTER, L., PHELPS, M., MAZZIOTA, J., *et al* (1987) Local cerebral glucose metabolic rates in obsessive–compulsive disorders. *Archives of General Psychiatry*, **44**, 211–218.
——— , SCHWARTZ, J., MAZZIOTTA, J., *et al* (1988) Cerebral glucose metabolic rates in non-depressed obsessive–compulsives. *American Journal of Psychiatry*, **145**, 1560–1563.
——— , ——— , BERGMAN, K., *et al* (1992) Caudate glucose metabolic rate changes with both drug and behavior therapy for obsessive–compulsive disorder. *Archives of General Psychiatry*, **49**, 681–689.
BENKELFAT, C., NORDHAL, T., SEMPLE, W., *et al* (1990) Local cerebral glucose metabolic rates in obsessive–compulsive disorder. *Archives of General Psychiatry*, **47**, 840–848.
CLOMIPRAMINE COLLABORATIVE GROUP (1991) Clomipramine in patients with obsessive compulsive disorder. *Archives of General Psychiatry*, **48**, 730–738.
COTTRAUX, J., MOLLARD, E., BOUVARD, M., *et al* (1990) A controlled study of fluvoxamine and exposure in obsessive–compulsive disorder. *International Clinical Psychopharmacology*, **5**, 17–20.
——— , ——— , ——— , *et al* (1993) Exposure therapy; fluvoxamine or combination treatment in obsessive–compulsive disorder: one year follow-up. *Psychiatry Research*, **49**, 63–75.
——— , CINOTTI, L., DEIBER, M. P., *et al* (1992) Testing cognitive theory of obsessive-compulsive disorder with PET-scan. Is it possible? Presented at World Congress of Cognitive Therapy, Toronto.
——— , MESSY, P., MARKS, I., *et al* (1993) Predictive factors in the treatment of obsessive-compulsive disorders with fluvoxamine and/or behaviour therapy. *Behavioural Psychotherapy*, **21**, 45–50.
EMMELKAMP, P., VAN DER HELM, M., VAN ZANTEN, B., *et al* (1980) Contribution of self-instructional training to the effectiveness of exposure *in vivo*: a comparison with obsessive-compulsive patients. *Behaviour Research and Therapy*, **18**, 61–66.
——— , VISSER, S. & HOEKSTRA, R. J. (1988) Cognitive therapy versus exposure *in vivo* in the treatment of obsessive–compulsive patients. *Cognitive Therapy and Research*, **12**, 103–114.
——— & BEENS, H. (1991) Cognitive therapy with obsessive–compulsive disorders: a comparative evaluation. *Behaviour Research and Therapy*, **29**, 293–300.
FOA, E., STEKETEE, G. & KOZAK, M. (1992) Treatment of depressive and obsessive-compulsive symptoms in obsessive-compulsive disorder by imipramine and behavior therapy. *British Journal of Clinical Psychology*, **31**, 279–292.
FREESTON, M. J., LADOUCEUR, R., THIBODEAU, H., *et al* (1991) Cognitive intrusions in non-clinical population. I. Response style, subjective experience and appraisal. *Behaviour Research and Therapy*, **29**, 585–597.
GOODMAN, W. K., PRICE, L. H., RASMUSSEN, S. A., *et al* (1989) Efficacy of fluvoxamine in obsessive–compulsive disorder. A double-blind comparison with placebo. *Archives of General Psychiatry*, **46**, 36–44.

GREIST, J., CHOUINARD, G., DUBOFF, E., *et al* (1992) Long-term sertraline treatment of obsessive–compulsive disorder: a 52-week double-blind comparative study versus placebo. *European Neuropsychopharmacology*, **3**, 386.

ILAI, G., SHOYER, B. & FOA, E. (1991) The effects of stimuli specificity and clinical severity on information processing in obsessive compulsive patients. Poster presented at the Association for the Advancement of Behavior Therapy, New York, November 22.

MACHLIN, S., HARRIS, G., PEARLSON, G., *et al* (1991) Elevated medial-frontal cerebral blood flow in obsessive–compulsive patients: a SPECT study. *American Journal of Psychiatry*, **148**, 1240–1242.

MARKS, I. (1987) *Fears, Phobias and Rituals: Panic, Anxiety, and their Disorders.* Oxford: Oxford University Press.

——, STERN, R. S., MAWSON, D., *et al* (1980) Clomipramine & exposure for obsessive–compulsive rituals. *British Journal of Psychiatry*, **136**, 1–25.

——, LELLIOTT, P., BASOGLU, M., *et al* (1988) Clomipramine, self-exposure and therapist-aided exposure in obsessive–compulsive ritualisers. *British Journal of Psychiatry*, **152**, 522–534.

MARTINOT, J. L., ALLILAIRE, J. F., MAZOYER, B. M., *et al* (1990) Obsessive–compulsive disorder: a clinical, neuropsychological and positron emission tomography study. *Acta Psychiatrica Scandinavica*, **82**, 233–242.

MINDUS, P., NYMAN, H., MOGARD, J., *et al* (1989) Orbital and caudate glucose metabolism studied by positron emission tomography (PET) in patients undergoing capsulotomy for obsessive compulsive disorder. In *Understanding Obsessive Compulsive Disorder (OCD)* (eds M. Jenike & M. Ashberg), pp. 52–57. Toronto: Hogrefe & Huber.

MONTEIRO, W., LELLIOTT, P., MARKS, I., *et al* (1986) Anorgasmia from clomipramine, in obsessive–compulsive disorder. *British Journal of Psychiatry*, **151**, 107–112.

MONTGOMERY, S. (1992) Are low doses effective in obsessive–compulsive disorder? Evidence from placebo controlled studies. *European Neuropsychopharmacology*, **3**, 199–200.

NILER, E. B. & BECK, S. J. (1989) The relationship among guilt dysphoria, anxiety and obsessions in a normal population. *Behaviour Research and Therapy*, **27**, 213–220.

NORDHAL, T., BENKELFAT, C., SEMPLE, W., *et al* (1989) Cerebral glucose metabolic rates in obsessive compulsive disorder. *Neuropsychopharmacology*, **2**, 1–7.

RACHMAN, S. & DE SILVA, P. (1978) Abnormal and normal obsessions. *Behaviour Research and Therapy*, **16**, 233–248.

REYNOLDS, M. & SALKOVSKIS, P. (1991) The relation among guilt anxiety and obsessions in a normal population. An attempted replication. *Behaviour Research and Therapy*, **29**, 259–265.

SALKOVSKIS, P. (1985) Obsessional–compulsive problems: a cognitive–behavioural analysis. *Behaviour Research and Therapy*, **23**, 571–583.

—— & HARRISON, J. (1984) Abnormal and normal obsessions – a replication. *Behaviour Research and Therapy*, **22**, 549–552.

SAWLE, G. V., HYMAS, N. F., LEES, A., *et al* (1991) Obsessional slowness. Functional studies with positron emission tomography. *Brain*, **114**, 2191–2202.

SOLYOM, L. & SOOKMAN, D. (1977) A comparison of clomipramine hydrochloride (Anafranil) and behaviour therapy in the treatment of obsessive–compulsive neurosis. *Journal of Internal Medicine Research*, **5** (suppl. 5), 49–61.

STERN, R., MARKS, I., MAWSON, D., *et al* (1980) Clomipramine and exposure for compulsive rituals: II. Plasma levels, side effects and outcome. *British Journal of Psychiatry*, **136**, 161–166.

SWEDO, S., SCHAPIRO, M., GRADY, C., *et al* (1989) Cerebral glucose metabolism in childhood onset obsessive–compulsive disorder. *Archives of General Psychiatry*, **46**, 518–523.

ZOHAR, J., INSEL, T., FOA, E., *et al* (1989) Physiological and psychological changes during *in vivo* exposure and imaginal flooding of obsessive compulsive disorder patients. *Archives of General Psychiatry*, **46**, 505–510.

11 Family interventions in schizophrenia

VLASSIS TOMARAS

Theories about the interactional causation of schizophrenia, implicating aberrant patterns of communication in the family that antedate the onset of the disorder, such as the 'double bind' hypothesis (Bateson *et al*, 1956), were formulated in the 1950s. Yet it was not possible for them to be tested; besides, they were thought to induce guilt in the relatives and therefore hamper their engagement in treatment.

Later, attention was refocused on family life, but this time as a factor associated with the course of schizophrenia. Some important reasons were:

(a) Improved medication strategies, and a mental health policy favouring the release of hospitalised patients to the community, rendering the family a frontline carer with the responsibility for their ill relative.

(b) Despite maintenance medication, even by parenteral administration, more than a third of patients relapsed in the first year after hospital discharge (Hogarty *et al*, 1974, 1979).

(c) An early study of Brown *et al* (1958) found that patients who lived with wives and parents showed a higher readmission rate than those going to brothers, sisters, more distant kin or lodgings.

Expressed emotion

Emotional atmosphere in the family has been successfully quantified by the use of 'expressed emotion' (EE), which measures attitudes and feelings of a relative toward the patient. Ratings of EE are made by a tape recorded, semistructured interview with the relative alone, known as the Camberwell Family Interview (CFI; Vaughn & Leff, 1976a). This is usually administered shortly after the patient has been admitted to hospital. Three out of the five scales of EE, namely the criticism, emotional overinvolvement and hostility scales, have been found to be predictive of relapse. A household is rated high on EE when any member scores above the cutoff on any of the three scales.

Regarding the construct validity of EE, the question has been posed as to whether it is simply an attitudinal index or an interactional one. Miklowitz *et al* (1984) provided evidence for significant correlation between EE and affective style (AS) codes, the latter being a coding system based on remarks made by the parent(s) to the patient during an actual, face-to-face discussion (Doane *et al*, 1981). Thus it can be argued that EE reflects, approximately, the interactional family process.

The predictive validity of EE has been adequately tested by 'naturalistic' studies, which demonstrated that relapse rates during the nine months after hospital discharge were significantly higher among schizophrenic patients returning to high-EE families than those to low-EE families. Relapse rates reported in three Anglo-American studies (Brown *et al*, 1972; Vaughn & Leff, 1976*b*; Vaughn *et al*, 1984) are 58 v. 16%, 50 v. 12% and 56 v. 17% respectively. Almost all replication studies so far, even across different cultures, have reached similar results.

The association between EE status and relapse can be interpreted in the context of the vulnerability–stress model of schizophrenia (Neuchterlein & Dawson, 1984), according to which there is an interaction between individual vulnerability factors and environmental stressors. Vulnerability factors include dopaminergic dysfunctions, abnormalities in attentional functioning and information processing, autonomic nervous system hyperactivity, and schizotypal personality traits. Environmental potentiators and stressors refer to a critical or emotionally overinvolved family climate, to an overstimulating social environment, and to stressful life-events. Excessive environmental stress, even in the presence of antipsychotic medication, may lead to a loss of balance and to 'intermediate states' (processing capacity overload, tonic autonomic hyperarousal, and deficient processing of social stimuli), finally resulting in a schizophrenic episode.

In a psychophysiological study by Tarrier *et al* (1979) in which skin conductance of schizophrenic patients in remission was measured, it was found that levels of arousal decreased when the patients interacted with a low-EE relative, whereas this was not evident with high-EE relatives. Their finding, which was interpreted as inability of arousal levels to habituate in stressful environments, is congruent with the observation in early EE studies (Vaughn & Leff, 1976*b*) that the amount of face-to-face interaction with high EE increases the risk of relapse.

Although the vulnerability–stress model is helpful for understanding how the adverse family environment precipitates schizophrenic episodes, mediating factors remain unclarified.

Family intervention studies

The predictive studies of EE gave impetus to controlled intervention studies, their goal being twofold: (a) to prevent relapse by decreasing the EE level, and to support family members, alleviate their burden, reduce tension, and enhance their coping and problem-solving skills; and (b) to further investigate the association between EE and relapse or the role of other family functioning factors in the course of schizophrenia. Despite the different concepts and methods employed in this series of studies, there is a common denominator which can be summarised as follows: EE is used as the selection criterion for high-risk families; they are engaged in treatment after hospital discharge; the experimental condition comprises family intervention, while controls receive routine or individual psychosocial treatment; both conditions are superimposed on regular antipsychotic medication; blindness is taken into consideration; assessments are made up to a two-year follow-up; family intervention, rather than traditional family therapy, has been readjusted to a version which is more structured, patient-centred and time-limited, accepting the reality of illness and providing information about it. The relevant studies published so far and their results regarding the patients are briefly reviewed here.

Positive results

Leff *et al* (1982, 1985) engaged 24 chronic schizophrenic patients, who were in high contact with high-EE relatives, in a controlled trial. Half the families were assigned to routine out-patient treatment, and the other half received a package of interventions which lasted nine months and consisted of: four lectures on the aetiology, symptomatology, course and treatment of schizophrenia; a relatives' group (21 sessions); family sessions in the home, which included the patient and varied in frequency according to the family's needs (ranging from 1 to 25). Their therapeutic approach was an eclectic one, combining educational, behavioural, structural and systemic techniques. They found a significant difference in relapse rates between the experimental and the control group (9% v. 50%) over nine months. The difference remained significant over the two-year follow-up assessment (20% v. 78%).

In the Falloon *et al* (1982, 1985, 1987) study, 36 patients participated, most of them belonging to high-EE households. The control treatment was individual supportive psychotherapy, while the family treatment consisted of 25 sessions conducted at home with the whole family. Although two sessions were devoted to psychoeducation, their 'family management' approach put emphasis on behavioural training in problem-solving and communication skills. The relapse rate for family-treated patients was 6%, compared with 44% for individually treated patients at the end of nine months of treatment. Significant advantages of family management were noted for symptom severity, community tenure, and social functioning. This reduced morbidity was sustained throughout the second year of follow-up.

Hogarty *et al* (1986) employed three experimental conditions in their two-year aftercare study: family treatment and medication; social skills training and medication; and their combination. All 90 treatment-takers lived in high-EE households. The psychoeducational family treatment, structured in four phases, included a 'survival skills workshop' (i.e. delivery of information in a multiple-family, day-long session in the absence of patients), as well as individual family sessions held over several months, focusing on specific management strategies, reinforcement of family boundaries and gradual resumption of responsibility by the patient (Anderson, 1986). First year relapse rates demonstrated important effects for family treatment (19%), for social skills training (20%) and an additive effect for the combined treatments (no relapses), relative to sole drug treatment (41%). Hogarty *et al* (1991) presented relapse data for the 90 treatment-takers at two years: 29% for the family treatment condition; 50% for the social skills training condition; 25% for the combined treatments; and 62% for the drug control condition. Their data suggest that the significant effect of family intervention on forestalling relapse persisted, whereas the additive effect of combined treatment had declined by two years.

Tarrier *et al* (1988, 1989) allocated 64 high-EE and 19 low-EE patients into four intervention groups: behavioural intervention enactive; behavioural intervention symbolic; education only; and routine treatment. Apart from the two educational sessions that all experimental groups experienced, there were 11 behavioural intervention sessions to teach skills for illness management. Symbolic intervention used symbolic representation such as discussion and instruction, whereas enactive intervention employed techniques such as role-playing, guided practice and record-keeping. Relapse rates at the end of the nine-month intervention period were significantly lower for patients in the enactive behavioural (17%) and the symbolic behavioural intervention (8%), compared with education only (43%) and routine treatment (53%) groups. In addition, patients who received family intervention showed considerable improvements in social functioning and activities compared with the high-EE control group (Barrowclough & Tarrier, 1990). According to the two-year assessment, the relapse rate of the behavioural family intervention group altogether was the same as the low-EE group (33%) and was significantly lower than that of the non-intervention high-EE group (59%). Tarrier *et al* (1989) suggested, on the basis of the data, that family intervention is able to delay relapse, but without continued intervention the risk of relapse is high.

In their second intervention study, Leff *et al* (1989, 1990), searching for the most effective component of the intervention package, compared education plus family therapy with education plus a relatives group. The study design was very similar to the first trial, and the sample was quite small ($n = 23$). The relapse rate over nine months in the family sessions group did not differ significantly from that of compliant families in the relatives sessions group (8% v. 17%). Patients' social functioning showed small, non-significant improvements. The relapse rates in the two groups were very much alike at two years (33% and 36% respectively).

Negative results

Kottgen *et al* (1984) used separate relative and patient groups. Their intervention was developed on an eclectic–psychodynamic basis; information was delivered in a less structured way. Neither continuous medication nor group therapy specifically affected the nine-month relapse rates (see Vaughn, 1986).

Vaughan *et al* (1992) carried out a controlled trial on 36 patients living in high-EE parental households. The parents of patients allocated to the intervention were offered ten counselling sessions. Relapses in the intervention group, although fewer, were not significantly different from the control group at nine months. The authors assumed that the exclusion of patients from the intervention, its short duration, and the lack of any involvement of the research team in patient care might have accounted for their results.

Other results

The Nithsdale schizophrenia surveys (McCreadie *et al*, 1991) offer an example of relatives' unwillingness to participate in a family intervention programme when patients are in remission. This might not be the rule, however, as indicated by a preliminary report by our team (Tomaras *et al*, 1990). Almost all high-EE relatives of chronic schizophrenics in remission living in the community, allocated to the intervention group, were involved in the relatives' group sessions.

Some studies which did not use the EE index are also noteworthy. Goldstein *et al* (1978) carried out a pioneering six-week controlled trial with young, mostly first-admission schizophrenics, and their families. A crisis-oriented, six-session family therapy strategy was adopted with four main objectives: identifying stressors; developing strategies both to avoid and cope with stress; implementing these strategies; anticipating and planning for future stressful experiences (Goldstein & Kopeikin, 1981). The data supported the combined prophylactic effects of an adequate dose of long-acting phenothiazine and family intervention in reducing relapse over six months.

Glick *et al* (1990) have reported on a psychoeducational family intervention applied during the in-patient phase of treatment. They noticed a favourable effect in terms of overall severity of illness and functioning in the family, although limited to women and impaired patients (with poor prehospital functioning).

There have been indications that psychodynamic, focal family therapy and supportive, problem-solving treatment can be equally effective, in terms of social functioning and community tenure (Levene *et al*, 1989). Key concepts in this brief therapy are the 'focal issue' and the 'focal change', the former consisting of the patient's regression, the parents' regressive behaviour toward him and their predisposition to their regression (i.e. passivity or immobilisation in the face of the patient's disturbed behaviour). Levene *et al* (1990) believe that this model could be reserved for families unable to benefit sufficiently from psychoeducation.

Components of intervention

Psychoeducation has generally been used as part of larger psychosocial interventions. This is based both on ethical grounds (the consumer should have access to information) and on grounds of therapeutic expediency (acquisition of knowledge should facilitate behavioural changes). Psychoeducation alone was found to be ineffective on relapse rates (Tarrier *et al*, 1988), but some beneficial effects have been reported. Cozolino *et al* (1988) noticed an increased sense of understanding of the illness and increased feelings of support from the treatment team for high-EE relatives after a single session of family education. However, they found no information retention after two months. Smith & Birchwood (1987) found that relatives' reported stress symptoms and fear of the patient were reduced after a four-session educational intervention; six months later, only knowledge gains and reduced perception of family burden had been maintained. Birchwood *et al* (1992) observed augmented gains in their recent study; there was increased optimism as to the family's role in treatment, reduction in relatives' stress and improvement in social functioning over six months.

Nonetheless, evidence has been provided that the shorter the length of illness, the more receptive relatives are to acquiring information (Barrowclough *et al*, 1987). A proportion of relatives tend to retain their own idiosyncratic beliefs about causes of the illness in spite of education (Berkowitz *et al*, 1984). It seems that recipients of information do not learn *ex vacuum*, but rather with pre-existing concepts and cognitive sets shaped over time. Tarrier & Barrowclough (1986), advocating the 'interaction model', put forward some guidelines: psychoeducation providers should assess and take seriously the relatives' views about the nature of schizophrenia and its management, before presenting alternative explanations and ways of coping. Information should be selective and focused on the particular patient's symptomatology. Also, the sooner information is delivered after the onset of illness, the more likely it is for individualised lay models of illness to be influenced.

Family sessions including the patient have been compared with relatives' sessions, and their efficacy in reducing relapse rate was found to be quite similar (Leff *et al*, 1990), although the non-compliance rate in the relatives' sessions group was high in this study. The former mode of intervention, if adopted in clinical practice, requires considerable professional resources. Evidence that the patient contributes to the negative escalation in the family suggests that he should participate in family intervention sessions (Hahlweg *et al*, 1987). Leff *et al* (1990) proposed that relatives' groups should be established in conjunction with some family sessions in the home.

Modification of familial factors

The studies in which the relatives' EE was reassessed at the end of the intervention indicated that significantly more reversals from high to low EE occurred in the experimental compared with the control group (Leff *et al*, 1982, 1989; Hogarty *et al*, 1986; Tarrier *et al*, 1988). Leff *et al* (1989) concluded that lowering of the relapse rate was mediated by a reduction in relatives' EE and/or face-to-face contact, and that it could not be explained by better compliance with medication. Nevertheless, data from these studies do not entirely support the causal role of EE in schizophrenic relapse.

Falloon *et al* (1986) argued that the benefits of behavioural family treatment mainly result from the improved capacity of families to cope with environmental stresses, and in particular with problem-solving situations. Family treatment in their study significantly reduced the negative affective climate of the family, and increased the parental ability to talk constructively with the patient during an emotionally charged discussion (Doane *et al*, 1986). Yet the nature of association between these changes and the acquisition of problem-solving skills by family members is not quite clear.

Conclusions

To date, research has shed light on the role of family stressors in schizophrenic relapse and course of the illness; questions such as how the patient perceives an adverse family environment and how he responds to it, or issues concerning the interaction of variables mediating recidivism, remain potential areas for further research.

The results of most intervention studies argue for routine family intervention in the community care of schizophrenia. This treatment modality could support long-term patients and their families, enhance their coping skills, improve the quality of family life and prevent clinical deterioration, in conjunction with medication and existing psychosocial rehabilitation programmes. In the case of overloaded mental health facilities, low-key family interventions combining support with psychoeducation (MacCarthy *et al*, 1989; Kuipers *et al*, 1989), which are practicable and less time-consuming, might be implemented.

References

ANDERSON, C. M. (1986) Psychoeducational family therapy. In *Treatment of Schizophrenia: Family Assessment and Intervention* (eds M. J. Goldstein, I. Hand & K. Hahlweg). Berlin: Springer-Verlag.
BARROWCLOUGH, C., TARRIER, N., WATTS, S., *et al* (1987) Assessing the functional value of relatives' knowledge about schizophrenia: a preliminary report. *British Journal of Psychiatry*, **151**, 1–8.

—— & —— (1990) Social functioning in schizophrenic patients: the effects of expressed emotion and family intervention. *Social Psychiatry and Psychiatric Epidemiology*, **25**, 125–129.

BATESON, G., JACKSON, D., HALEY, J., *et al* (1956) Toward a theory of schizophrenia. *Behavioral Science*, **1**, 252–264.

BERKOWITZ, R., EBERLEIN-VRIES, R., KUIPERS, L., *et al* (1984) Educating relatives about schizophrenia. *Schizophrenia Bulletin*, **10**, 418–429.

BIRCHWOOD, M., SMITH, J. & COCHRANE, R. (1992) Specific and non-specific effects of educational intervention for families living with schizophrenia. A comparison of three methods. *British Journal of Psychiatry*, **160**, 806–814.

BROWN, G. W., CARSTAIRS, G. M. & TOPPING, G. D. (1958) Post-hospital adjustment of chronic mental patients. *Lancet*, **2**, 685–689.

——, BIRLEY, J. L. T. & WING, J. K. (1972) Influence of family life on the course of schizophrenic disorders: a replication. *British Journal of Psychiatry*, **121**, 241–258.

COZOLINO, L. J., GOLDSTEIN, M. J., NUECHTERLEIN, K. H., *et al* (1988) The impact of education about schizophrenia on relatives varying in expressed emotion. *Schizophrenia Bulletin*, **14**, 675–687.

DOANE, J. A., WEST, K. L., GOLDSTEIN, M. J., *et al* (1981) Parental communication deviance and affective style: predictors of subsequent schizophrenia spectrum disorders in vulnerable adolescents. *Archives of General Psychiatry*, **38**, 679–685.

——, GOLDSTEIN, M. J., MIKLOWITZ, D. J., *et al* (1986) The impact of individual and family treatment on the affective climate of families of schizophrenics. *British Journal of Psychiatry*, **148**, 279–287.

FALLOON, I. R. H., BOYD, J. L., McGILL, C. W., *et al* (1982) Family management in the prevention of exacerbations of schizophrenia: a controlled study. *New England Journal of Medicine*, **306**, 1437–1440.

——, ——, ——, *et al* (1985) Family management in the prevention of morbidity of schizophrenia: clinical outcome of a two-year longitudinal study. *Archives of General Psychiatry*, **42**, 887–896.

——, PEDERSON, J. & AL-KHAYYAL, M. (1986) Enhancement of health-giving family support versus treatment of family pathology. *Journal of Family Therapy*, **8**, 339–350.

——, McGILL, C. W., BOYD, J. L., *et al* (1987) Family management in the prevention of morbidity of schizophrenia: social outcome of a two-year longitudinal study. *Psychological Medicine*, **17**, 59–66.

GLICK, I. D., SPENCER, J. H., CLARKIN, J. F., *et al* (1990) A randomized clinical trial of inpatient family intervention: IV. Follow-up results for subjects with schizophrenia. *Schizophrenia Research*, **3**, 187–200.

GOLDSTEIN, M. J., RODNICK, E. H., EVANS, J. R., *et al* (1978) Drug and family therapy in the aftercare of acute schizophrenics. *Archives of General Psychiatry*, **35**, 1169–1177.

—— & KOPEIKIN, H. S. (1981) Short- and long-term effects of combining drug and family therapy. In *New Directions for Mental Health Services: New Developments in Interventions with Families of Schizophrenics* (ed. M. Goldstein). San Francisco: Jossey-Bass.

HAHLWEG, K., NUECHTERLEIN, K. H., GOLDSTEIN, M. J., *et al* (1987) Parental expressed emotion attitudes and intrafamilial communication behavior. In *Understanding Major Mental Disorder. The Contribution of Family Interaction Research* (eds K. Hahlweg & M. J. Goldstein). New York: Family Process Press.

HOGARTY, G. E., GOLDBERG, S. C., SCHOOLER, N. R., *et al* (1974) Drug and sociotherapy in the aftercare of schizophrenic patients. *Archives of General Psychiatry*, **31**, 603–608.

——, SCHOOLER, N. R., ULRICH, R., *et al* (1979) Fluphenazine and social therapy in the aftercare of schizophrenic patients. *Archives of General Psychiatry*, **36**, 1283–1294.

——, ANDERSON, C. M., REISS, D. J., *et al* (1986) Family psychoeducation, social skills training and maintenance chemotherapy in the aftercare treatment of schizophrenia. *Archives of General Psychiatry*, **43**, 633–642.

——, ——, ——, *et al* (1991) Family psychoeducation, social skills training and maintenance chemotherapy in the aftercare treatment of schizophrenia: II. Two-year effects of a controlled study on relapse and adjustment. *Archives of General Psychiatry*, **48**, 340–347.

KOTTGEN, C., SONNICHSEN, I., MOLLENHAUER, K., *et al* (1984) Results of the Hambourg Camberwell Family Interview Study, I–III. *International Journal of Family Psychiatry*, **5**, 61–94.

KUIPERS, L., MACCARTHY, B., HURRY, J., *et al* (1989) Counselling the relatives of the long-term adult mentally ill: II. A low-cost supportive model. *British Journal of Psychiatry*, **154**, 775–782.

LEFF, J., KUIPERS, L., BERKOWITZ, R., *et al* (1982) A controlled trial of social intervention in the families of schizophrenic patients. *British Journal of Psychiatry*, **141**, 121–134.

——, ——, ——, *et al* (1985) A controlled trial of social intervention in the families of schizophrenic patients: two year follow-up. *British Journal of Psychiatry*, **146**, 594–600.

——, BERKOWITZ, R., SHAVIT, N., *et al* (1989). A trial of family therapy v. a relatives group for schizophrenia. *British Journal of Psychiatry*, **154**, 58–66.

——, ——, ——, *et al* (1990) A trial of family therapy versus a relatives' group for schizophrenia: two-year follow-up. *British Journal of Psychiatry*, **157**, 571–577.

LEVENE, J. E., NEWMAN, F. & JEFFERIES, J. J. (1989) Focal family therapy outcome study, I: Patient and family functioning. *Canadian Journal of Psychiatry*, **34**, 641–647.

——, —— & —— (1990) Focal family therapy: theory and practice. *Family Process*, **29**, 73–86.

MACCARTHY, B., KUIPERS, L., HURRY, J., *et al* (1989) Counselling the relatives of the long-term adult mentally ill, I. Evaluation of the impact on relatives and patients. *British Journal of Psychiatry*, **154**, 768–775.

MCCREADIE, R. G., PHILLIPS, K., HARVEY, J. A., *et al* (1991) The Nithsdale schizophrenia surveys. VIII: Do relatives want family intervention – and does it help? *British Journal of Psychiatry*, **158**, 110–113.

MIKLOWITZ, D. J., GOLDSTEIN, M. J., FALLOON, R. H., *et al* (1984) Interactional correlates of expressed emotion in the families of schizophrenics. *British Journal of Psychiatry*, **144**, 482–487.

NUECHTERLEIN, K. H. & DAWSON, M. H. (1984) A heuristic vulnerability/stress model of schizophrenic episodes. *Schizophrenia Bulletin*, **10**, 300–312.

SMITH, J. V. & BIRCHWOOD, M. J. (1987) Specific and non-specific effects of educational intervention with families living with a schizophrenic relative. *British Journal of Psychiatry*, **150**, 645–652.

TARRIER, N., VAUGHN, C. E., LADER, M. H., *et al* (1979) Bodily reactions to people and events in schizophrenia. *Archives of General Psychiatry*, **36**, 311–315.

—— & BARROWCLOUGH, C. (1986) Providing information to relatives about schizophrenia: some comments. *British Journal of Psychiatry*, **149**, 458–463.

——, ——, VAUGHN, C., *et al* (1988). The community management of schizophrenia: a controlled trial of a behavioural intervention with families to reduce relapse. *British Journal of Psychiatry*, **153**, 532–542.

——, ——, ——, *et al* (1989) Community management of schizophrenia: a two-year follow-up of a behavioural intervention with families. *British Journal of Psychiatry*, **154**, 625–628.

TOMARAS, V., KARYDI, V., MAVREAS, V., *et al* (1990) Expressed emotion: risk and protective factors in schizophrenia relapse in Greece. In *Psychiatry: A World Perspective*, vol. 3 (eds C. N. Stefanis, A. D. Rabavilas & C. R. Soldatos). Amsterdam: Excerpta Medica.

VAUGHAN, K., DOYLE, M., MCCONAGHY, N., *et al* (1992) The Sydney intervention trial: a controlled trial of relatives' counselling to reduce schizophrenic relapse. *Social Psychiatry and Psychiatric Epidemiology*, **27**, 16–21.

VAUGHN, C. (1986) Comment on chapter 5. In *Treatment of Schizophrenia: Family Assessment and Intervention* (eds M. J. Goldstein, I. Hand & K. Hahlweg). Berlin: Springer-Verlag.

—— & LEFF, J. (1976a) The measurement of expressed emotion in families of psychiatric patients. *British Journal of Social and Clinical Psychology*, **15**, 157–165.

—— & —— (1976b) The influence of family and social factors on the course of psychiatric illness. *British Journal of Psychiatry*, **129**, 125–137.

——, SNYDER, K. S., JONES, S., *et al* (1984) Family factors in schizophrenic relapse. *Archives of General Psychiatry*, **41**, 1169–1177.

12 Counselling for families of children with chronic disabilities

HILTON DAVIS

This chapter is intended as a respectful tribute to the ability of children and their families to cope with the adversity of chronic disease and disability over many years. Although the focus is on intervention strategies for families of children with disabilities, the points made apply to all families with children with chronic diseases. The overall message is:

> The effectiveness of help for children with chronic disease and disability is likely to be reduced unless careful attention is given to the psychosocial adaptation of parents, and therefore intervention has to be broadly based, family-oriented and preventive.

This message has yet to be properly heard in the UK, and is applicable to all states, not only in the European Union but internationally.

This chapter reviews the psychosocial effects of chronic disease and disability on families, before considering the dominant model of early intervention in the area of intellectual disability. The effectiveness of this model will then be reviewed, leading on to a consideration of alternative models, the kind of service to be derived from them, and available evaluative evidence.

Psychosocial effects of chronic disability

The disclosure of a serious diagnosis is a major crisis for parents and their children, and sets in motion processes of adaptation that frequently lead to major changes in the life of the family, and potentially serious psychological and social disturbance (Eiser, 1990a,b).

For the children, there is a two- to three-fold increase in behavioural and emotional problems. Where there is both disease and disability, more than 30% of children may show such disturbance (Cadman et al, 1987). Cognitive and academic problems are frequent accompaniments of the physical

125

problems (Garrison & McQuiston, 1989), and there is evidence that psychological disturbance is associated with poor compliance with treatment (Garralda *et al*, 1988).

Parents not only have to cope with the disability or disease and the emotional pain this brings (Van Dongen-Melman & Sanders-Woudstra, 1986), but they also have to deal with the emotional problems of the child, and they are frequently involved in direct educational activities (Cunningham, 1985). Increased time, energy, attention, and financial demands are therefore made on parents, and it is not surprising that problems may arise. Parents may be fatigued and have financial difficulties (Burr, 1986; Satterwhite, 1978). There may be less time for themselves, for leisure and relaxation, for family activities as a whole, or for career pursuit. Studies frequently indicate increased parental stress (Johnson, 1985) and psychological disturbance, including anxiety, depression and communication difficulties (Shapiro, 1983; Hughes & Lieberman, 1990). For example, in a recently completed (as yet unpublished) study of mothers of children with diabetes, the Parenting Stress Index (Abidin, 1990) showed the mean for total stress to be at the 87th percentile compared to the normative sample, and that approximately 31% of the mothers were clinically anxious (Staples & Davis, 1993).

The situation for other members of the family has been less well documented, and the evidence is somewhat inconsistent. However, studies suggest that siblings are affected by the disease or disability (Van Dongen-Melman & Sanders-Woudstra, 1986; Burr, 1985; Johnson, 1985). Given that the family is a system, then disturbance in one member is bound to affect all the others (Shapiro, 1983), and there is evidence of lower cohesion, less open communication and more conflict in families (Eiser, 1990*a*), including increased marital disharmony (Sabbeth & Leventhal, 1984). However, although the effects of stress may be mitigated by good social support, parents may feel more isolated in the context of chronic disease (Walker *et al*, 1971; Shapiro, 1983).

These findings are not presented with the intention of emphasising pathology. Although most parents will be distressed at various times during the disease process, the majority adapt well. However, it should not be forgotten that the situation for families coping with disease and disability is highly stressful, that the process of adaptation takes time, and that it does affect all aspects of treatment (Davis & Fallowfield, 1991*a*). As such, the adaptation of all members of the family should be considered seriously at all times by health care personnel.

Current service intervention model

Services tend to be orientated towards the child, and more specifically towards his/her health and ability. In practice, the more general well-being of the child is not a priority, and few services take a broad family approach. There is certainly little concern for the prevention of adaptational problems, or to deal with them when they arise. Also, the rather poor communication skills exhibited by professionals (Davis & Fallowfield, 1991*b*) will not enhance family adaptation and may even hinder the process. There are, for example, high levels of parental dissatisfaction with the way in which diagnoses are disclosed (Cunningham *et al*, 1984; Jupp, 1992), and problems with communication are the biggest source of complaint about health care professionals in all areas of medicine (Ley, 1988).

Such findings are not surprising, given the usual model of service delivery in, for example, early intervention in the area of intellectual disability. The most common model is as follows:

(a) train professionals
(b) to teach parents
(c) to relate to, stimulate and/or educate their child appropriately
(d) in order to facilitate the child's development.

The emphasis is on the child, without consideration of parental adaptation or the professional skills required for this.

It is not surprising, therefore, that the evidence for the effectiveness of such early intervention is disappointing. In their review, Davis & Rushton (1991) found that although parents may be effective in changing specific child behaviours, their ability to produce short-term generalised developmental effects has not been shown conclusively, and long-term benefits of current intervention strategies have not been found (Cunningham, 1987). However, only rarely have researchers evaluated the effects upon parents themselves, and nor has a more broadly based theory been made explicit to take account of all family members.

An alternative

In order to set up an intervention system cogniscent of the many possible family difficulties, an attempt has been made to develop appropriate and explicit theoretical frameworks on which to base intervention. The conclusions are described in detail in Davis (1993). In contrast to the four-step model described earlier, the new model is as follows:

(a) train professionals
(b) in the basic skills of counselling
(c) to establish a partnership with parents,
(d) which would provide support,
(e) enhance parental self-esteem,

(f) allow parents to explore the whole problem facing them,
(g) help them adapt by reconstruing the situation clearly
(h) so as to set their own clear goal,
(i) to decide for themselves what to do,
(j) thus optimising the general family environment,
(k) thereby optimising the child's development as a whole.

The central concern is principally with the psychological adaptation of the parents, and secondly the children. The reality is that if, for whatever reason, parents are unable or do not want to follow professional advice in all its aspects, then available help for the child is minimised. This may be, for example, because of: preoccupation with other problems; personal psychological difficulties; not understanding the professional; conflicting aims; dissatisfaction with the professional; or mistrust of their advice.

Underlying this model are a number of frameworks to do with parental adaptation, the process of helping, the nature of the relationship, and the qualities of the helper. Each of these will be discussed briefly in turn.

Parental adaptation

This is understood in terms of the personal construct theory of George Kelly (1955). It is assumed that at diagnosis, the parent's model of the world (their construct system) is potentially invalidated in all respects. The information they are given is of such importance that it will possibly change their world in all its aspects. At the very least the validity of their existing construct system to the new situation will suddenly become unknown, and will have to be explored. It is the process of exploration and change that is the central factor in adaptation. The process includes learning about the illness or disability and associated services. However, parents' constructs about their child are likely to alter, as are their self-constructions, their constructs about their spouse/partner, their other children, extended family, friends, neighbours, their life situation more generally, including their work, finances, interests and home care. An important task is the exploration of the effect of the new situation upon their whole philosophy and meaning of life (e.g. religion and values).

The process of helping

This is conventionally seen as the professional providing limited knowledge about the disease/disability and its appropriate treatment. The view endorsed here is broader than this, and requires a framework for understanding the process of helping. Such a framework must encompass the sharing of technical knowledge and treatment advice, and can be conceptualised following the work of Egan (1986) as a number of tasks that are largely sequential. These are:

(a) establishment of an effective relationship
(b) exploration of the parent's perspective
(c) development of clear models
(d) negotiation of general aims and specific goals
(e) careful planning of appropriate strategies
(f) implementation of the plans
(g) evaluation of outcome.

This is simplified in that steps may be omitted, one might backtrack following evaluation, or work through the process several times for different problems. However, the first three tasks are particularly important in the context of conditions that are in essence incurable and likely to remain for the lifetime of the child. Establishing a close relationship in which parents feel respected is of enormous value to them in adapting to the situations confronting them. Its value lies in the increased self-esteem to be derived from such a relationship, but also because of the opportunity the relationship provides for the careful exploration of all aspects of the parents' personal and family situation.

The helping relationship

This is conceptualised as a partnership between the parent and professional, and is characterised as:

(a) working closely together
(b) establishing common aims
(c) acknowledgement of complementary expertise
(d) showing mutual respect
(e) skilled communication
(f) constant negotiation with or without conflict
(g) honesty
(h) flexibility.

Helper qualities

A number of important characteristics and skills are required of the professional to establish such a relationship, to carry out the tasks specified earlier, and hence to facilitate parental adaptation. These include five fundamental attitudes, related to the work of Rogers (1959), and a set of skills by which these are demonstrated. The attitudes include: respect, humility, genuineness, empathy, and quiet enthusiasm. Our framework suggests that these should be demonstrated in all aspects of professional behaviour, but particularly in relation to basic skills such as active attention to the parents, the skills of listening, the ability to foster the circumstances in which parents are prepared to talk openly, and the skills of exploring problems broadly.

The Parent Adviser Scheme

The Parent Adviser Scheme was set up with the Tower Hamlets Child Development Team in east London as a way of supporting families of children with intellectual and/or multiple disabilities. Existing professionals were trained on a course specially designed to discuss the models underlying the service (as above), and in the basic counselling skills necessary to carry out the work.

Once trained, the participants (parent advisers) were asked to see up to two families, and to visit them at home, initially weekly, and then as negotiated with each family at increasing intervals up to once a month, or in a crisis. The focus of the sessions was not necessarily the child, but whatever issues were of concern to the parents. Emphasis was given to establishing a partnership with parents as opposed to solving their problems. The major intention was to make parents feel good about themselves, to help them explore issues, decide their own aims, and enable them to use their own resources to best effect.

Since many of the families served by the Child Development Team were of Bangladeshi origin and mostly non-English speaking, the system would have been of little value without a Bangladeshi Parent Adviser. Fortunately, a generous grant from the Mental Health Foundation not only allowed us to employ a full-time Bangladeshi Parent Adviser, but also allowed us to evaluate the whole project.

Research evaluation

The service was set up with a built-in research component. This included evaluation of the training of the parent advisers, an evaluation of the intervention with English-speaking families, and an evaluation of the Bangladeshi service. The design of the service evaluations involved assessing families on a broad range of measures before and after intervention, with random allocation of families to intervention or control groups. Families in the control groups were assessed in the same way as those with the intervention, but received only the usual routine services. The study was conducted by a research psychologist funded by the Mental Health Foundation and independent of the clinical staff. Full details of the research can be found in Davis & Rushton (1991) and Rushton & Davis (1992).

Evaluation is difficult, especially in the context of complex theory and practice, as was the case in the present research. Nevertheless, the research to date has given considerable weight to the models proposed.

Mothers were assessed before and after the intervention, which lasted 15 months on average. The assessment was multifaceted, and many of the results were based on self-ratings using seven-point bipolar scales in repertory grid formats. The results indicated that not only did the mothers in the Parent Adviser group improve significantly over the time of the study, they also improved significantly more than the controls. The intervention group came to see themselves as much better supported in general, by professionals and non-professionals (friends, neighbours and family). These improvements in perceived social support were endorsed by a significant increase in the number of social contacts per year in the Parent Adviser group. There were improvements in the extent to which mothers felt involved by professionals in the child's treatment, in their ability to help their children, and in their joy in caring for their child. There were significant reductions in perceived stress. Mothers came to feel they neglected their other children less. There were highly significant improvements in the mother's self-esteem. They felt less depressed themselves, more positive towards their children, and more positive towards their husbands.

Given that the focus of the intervention was on the parents, the results indicated that the mothers had benefited significantly as predicted, and it could be inferred that the families were functioning better as a unit. This contrasts with the control group, which either showed no changes or deteriorated, providing some evidence that the intervention was preventive as well as ameliorative.

Although the children were not the primary focus of the intervention, nevertheless, as predicted, the children in the intervention group derived significant benefits compared to the controls. For example, there were highly significant reductions in behaviour problems in the intervention children, and significant increases in developmental level, despite the fact that they were all severely delayed globally.

Conclusions

These results provide empirical support for the contention that parental adaptation is a crucial variable in services for children, and that counselling is not only effective in helping parents to adapt to the situation of disability, but is also of direct benefit to their children, even when teaching is not the strategy employed. The findings further support the notion that a model of partnership between parent and professional is appropriate to the health care context, that a counselling model may serve as a guide for professional communication behaviour, and that the fundamental attitudes and basic skills of counselling are appropriate and beneficial to both parents, their families and children.

Research is needed to explore, evaluate and elaborate further the ideas presented here. The various studies need replication in relation to different disease categories, and more detailed questions need to be addressed. However, the current findings are sufficiently strong to indicate the value of intervention studies, particularly as there are so few studies of this type in paediatrics (e.g. Pless & Satterwhite, 1972; Stein & Jessop, 1984).

The results so far should not be taken to suggest that early intervention involving parents training their children is of no value, only that the value has yet to be demonstrated. However, the findings do suggest that any value to be derived from parent teaching will only occur if it is set in the context of good professional communication and support.

There are important implications for service development. Perhaps the most important is that highly specialist mental health professionals are not necessarily needed to work with families. The research suggests that all professionals, and even non-professional volunteers, can work effectively with families. Secondly, the reduced need for highly trained specialised personnel means that the possibility of helping ethnic minority groups, even those who cannot speak the language of the indigenous population, is increased enormously. With support from professionals, members of ethnic minority groups without previous professional education can be trained in a very short time in this intervention strategy. The system proposed here is applicable to different cultures and countries in Europe and further afield. The work presented here is currently being extended in the UK, where we have begun to work with a range of childhood problems, other racial groups, and in a variety of settings. A further study is currently being planned in Singapore.

References

ABIDIN, R. (1990) *Parenting Stress Index: Short Form*. Charlottesville, VA: Pediatric Psychology Press.

BURR, C. (1985) Impact on the family of a chronically ill child. In *Issues in the Care of Children with Chronic Illness* (eds N. Hobbs & J. Perrin). San Francisco: Jossey-Bass.

CADMAN, D., BOYLE, M., SZATMARI, P., *et al* (1987) Chronic illness, disability and mental and social well-being: findings of the Ontario Child Health Study. *Paediatrics*, **79**, 805–813.

CUNNINGHAM, C. (1985) Training and education approaches for parents of children with special needs. *British Journal of Medical Psychology*, **58**, 285–305.

—— (1987) Early intervention in Down's syndrome. In *Prevention of Mental Handicap: A World Review* (eds G. Hosking & G. Murphy). London: Royal Society of Medicine.

——, MORGAN, P. & McGUCKEN, R. (1984) Down's syndrome: is dissatisfaction with disclosure of diagnosis inevitable? *Developmental Medicine and Child Neurology*, **26**, 33–39.

DAVIS, H. (1993) *Counselling Parents of Children with Chronic Illness or Disability*. Leicester: British Psychological Society.

—— & FALLOWFIELD, L. (1991*a*) Evaluating the effects of counselling and communication. In *Counselling and Communication in Health Care* (eds H. Davis & L. Fallowfield). Chichester: John Wiley.

—— & —— (1991*b*) Counselling and communication in health care: the current situation. In *Counselling and Communication in Health Care* (eds H. Davis & L. Fallowfield). Chichester: John Wiley.

—— & RUSHTON, R. (1991) Counselling and supporting parents of children with developmental delay: a research evaluation. *Journal of Mental Deficiency Research*, **35**, 89–112.

EGAN, G. (1986) *The Skilled Helper*. Monterey: Brooks/Cole.

EISER, C. (1990*a*) *Chronic Childhood Disease*. Cambridge: Cambridge University Press.

—— (1990*b*) Psychological effects of chronic disease. *Journal of Child Psychology and Psychiatry*, **31**, 85–98.

GARRALDA, M., JAMESON, R., REYNOLDS, J., *et al* (1988) Psychiatric adjustment in children with chronic renal failure. *Journal of Child Psychology and Psychiatry*, **29**, 79–90.

GARRISON, W. & McQUISTON, S. (1989) *Chronic Illness During Childhood and Adolescence: Psychological Aspects*. New York: Sage.

HUGHES, P. & LIEBERMAN, S. (1990) Troubled parents: vulnerability and stress in childhood cancer. *British Journal of Medical Psychology*, **63**, 53–64.

JOHNSON, S. (1985) The family and the child with chronic illness. In *Health, Illness, and Families: A Life-span Perspective* (ed. D. Turk & R. Kerns). New York: John Wiley.

JUPP, S. (1992) *Congenital Anomaly: Disclosure of Diagnosis and Early Support*. PhD thesis submitted to the University of Manchester.

KELLY, G. (1955) *The Psychology of Personal Constructs*. New York: Norton.

LEY, P. (1988) *Communicating with Patients: Improving Communication, Satisfaction and Compliance*. London: Croom Helm.

PLESS, I. & SATTERWHITE, B. (1972) Chronic illness in childhood: selection, activities and evaluation of non-professional family counselors. *Clinical Pediatrics*, **11**, 403–410.

ROGERS, C. (1959) A theory of therapy, personality, and interpersonal relationships, as developed in the client-centered framework. In *Psychology: A Study of a Science* (ed. S. Koch). New York: McGraw-Hill.

RUSHTON, R. & DAVIS, H. (1992) An evaluation of training in basic counselling skills. *British Journal of Guidance and Counselling*, **20**, 206–221.

SABBETH, B. & LEVENTHAL, J. (1984) Marital adjustment to chronic childhood illness: a critique of the literature. *Pediatrics*, **73**, 762–767.

SATTERWHITE, B. (1978) The impact of chronic illness on child and family: an overview based on five surveys with implications for management. *International Journal of Rehabilitative Research*, **1**, 1–17.

SHAPIRO, J. (1983) Family reactions and coping strategies in response to the physically ill or handicapped child: a review. *Social Science and Medicine*, **17**, 913–931.

STAPLES, E. & DAVIS, H. (1993) Parental adaptation in the context of childhood diabetes. In preparation.

STEIN, R. & JESSOP, D. (1984) Does pediatric home care make a difference for children with chronic illness? *Pediatrics*, **73**, 845–853.

VAN DONGEN-MELMAN, J. & SANDERS-WOUSTRA, J. (1986) Psychosocial aspects of childhood cancer: a review of the literature. *Journal of Child Psychology and Psychiatry*, **27**, 145–180.

WALKER, J., THOMAS, M. & RUSSELL, I. (1971) Spina bifida and the parents. *Developmental Medicine and Child Neurology*, **13**, 462–476.

Part V. Service delivery

13 Detaining psychiatric patients

LUCIA WHITNEY, PALOMA RUIZ
and MICHAEL LANGENBACH

Since the 18th century there have been a great variety of mental health laws as different countries have attempted to develop a legal framework for the compulsory admission and detention of psychiatric patients (Curran & Harding, 1978; Soothill *et al*, 1981; Soothill, 1990). There have been countless discussions about the implications of compulsory measures in psychiatry, the appropriateness of legislation, and the fairness of professional procedures throughout the world (Scull, 1984; Marschner, 1986; Rose, 1986; Smith, 1991). A recent stimulus to the discussion has been provided by the further development of the European Community (EC) and moves towards increasing harmonisation of legal arrangements. This chapter reviews current practice in parts of the EC. We have restricted our attention to civil commitments, without considering the provision for criminal psychiatric patients.

The current situation in Europe

There are substantial similarities among continental European practices, and important differences from the Mental Health Act of England & Wales (Department of Health and Social Security, 1984). These differences are mostly due to the different legal systems in the countries under consideration.

While continental Europe is mainly influenced by the Romano-Germanic legal tradition dating back to the *Corpus Iuris* of the Emperor Justinian, UK law is based on Common Law and the principles of Equity and is only slightly influenced by Roman Law (David & Jauffret Spinosi, 1988). Continental legislation is deductive and scholastically organised; each case is considered in relation to the whole system of legal principles. The individual problem is viewed in the abstract and resolved by reference to the terms of the Civil Code. The UK method, in contrast, is forensic, pragmatic and inductive looking for individual case solutions by inferring *de similibus ad similia*.

This pragmatic orientation of UK law has influenced the Mental Health Act 1983, as the systematic method has influenced the corresponding legislation on the continent.

We would like to describe the consequences of this legislative contrast by looking at the mental health laws in Germany, Italy and Spain. The UK legislation will be referred to in the discussion.

The legislation

In Germany, the detention of psychiatric patients is possible only as an exception from the basic human right of freedom of the person and freedom of movement guaranteed by articles 2, 11 and 104 of the *Grundgesetz* (constitution). These constitutional rights can be restricted only by legal measures enacted by a legally entitled person (Hesse, 1984). Accordingly, the detention of a person for psychiatric reasons is seen primarily as a legal problem, and can only be ordered by a judge after a court hearing.

As Germany is a federation, there is not yet a nationwide law for the involuntary detention of psychiatric patients, each state having its own law. The regional differences are, however, not significant, and are mainly procedural. In this study we consider the legislation of North Rhine–Westphalia which, with a population of over 15 million, is the biggest state of the federation. Here the detention of psychiatric patients is regulated by the *Gesetz uber Hilfen und Schutzmasnahmen bei Psychischen Krankheiten* (law concerning help and protection in psychiatric illnesses) of 1969 (Eberhard, 1980).

In Spain, compulsory admissions were regulated by the ''decreto'' of 3 June 1931, until the passing of Law 13/83 on 24 October 1983.

In Italy, the old law of 1904 was amended in 1968, but a new act was only established in 1978. This is the well-known Law 180.

Grounds

In Germany, patients are considered detainable when suffering from a psychosis or a psychiatric disorder with psychotic effects, or from addiction or mental handicap. However, they may only be detained when they cannot be helped in other ways and when they present a danger either to themselves (specifically the danger of suicide or self-harm) or to others. Although these dangers need to be acute, the law acknowledges the fact that behaviour is unpredictable, and the expectation of danger can be sufficient reason to detain a patient.

In Spain it is only necessary to recognise that the patient is a *presunto incapaz* (presumed incapable). A patient is presumed incapable by the legislation when suffering from a mental disorder (organic or functional), mental retardation or serious drug or alcohol addiction, and because of this disorder is unable to manage himself and his own affairs (Ortega-Monasterio, 1991).

In Italy, Law 180 states that measures for compulsory treatment can be taken in respect of persons suffering from mental disorder (no definition is given for mental disorder). The proposal for compulsory treatment can encompass hospitalisation only if the mental disturbance is such as to require urgent therapeutic intervention, if the patient refuses treatment, and if the conditions and circumstances for taking timely health care measures outside the hospital do not exist (Pizzi, 1978).

Application and certification

Application to detain a patient in Germany is made by the local *Ordnungsbehörde* (Town Clerk's Office). The decision to detain is then made by a judge after hearing the patient. A doctor (not necessarily a psychiatrist) fills the role of expert witness and has to provide certification of the patient's psychiatric state. In practice, doctors are often the initial source of application and they involve the town clerk to initiate the formal procedure.

In cases of acute danger, a patient can be detained immediately by the clerk's office. In this case, the patient must be seen by a judge before the end of the following day.

In Spain, application can be made by the patient's relatives, neighbours, teachers or any other interested party. Authorisation for compulsory admission is granted by a judge. For an emergency admission, the judge decides after seeing the application and in some circumstances asks for an assessment by a forensic doctor (*forense*). In normal circumstances the judge makes his decision after hearing the patient and a medical opinion (it is the judge who nominates the doctor).

Compulsory health treatment in Italy is ordered by a Mayor after a formal proposal from a doctor (usually the general practitioner), ratified by a public health service psychiatrist or other authorised health service doctor. Formal notice of this measure must be delivered to the district judge by local government messenger within 48 hours of admission. The judge then has two days to make any necessary enquiries and issue a decree confirming or overturning the measure. Neither the judge nor the Mayor hears the patient.

There is no statutory involvement of social workers in Germany, Spain or Italy.

Length of stay

In Germany, when the emergency admission procedure is used, the judge can detain the patient for an initial maximum of two months, either because it is expected that the detention will be of short duration, or to give time to prepare a detailed assessment of the patient's mental state. Longer periods of detention of up to six months can only be ordered by the judge after a detailed assessment by a psychiatrist. Repeats are possible. The detention has to be curtailed immediately the reasons for the detention are no longer present.

Detention includes the right to treat patients against their wishes, apart from treatments which carry a high health risk or which may cause significant personality changes. In such cases, either the patient or a specific medico-legal commission must give permission.

In Spain there is no time limit for the duration of the compulsory treatment, and it can vary enormously. The patient is discharged when he is considered well enough to leave the hospital. The compulsory treatment in Italy is only for seven days. It can be extended, and in this case the doctor responsible for the mental health service must send a formal request to the Mayor indicating the predicted further duration of the treatment. The Mayor then obtains the necessary decree from a judge. The doctor is obliged to notify the Major of the cessation of the conditions which required the compulsory admission (whether or not the patient remains in hospital). The Major must then inform the judge within 48 hours.

Other matters

In Germany and Spain there is no specific provision for appeal in the mental health legislation, but there is a right of appeal through the legal system.

In Italy, anyone who undergoes compulsory treatment and any other interested party can appeal against the judge's decree to the Court of his jurisdiction.

There are no provisions for compulsory treatment in the community in any of these countries, but detention does include the right to treat patients against their wishes.

Comparison with the UK

The most notable similarity between the regulations covering compulsory admissions in Germany, Italy and Spain is the obligatory authorisation of these measures by a judge. In Italy, however, because of the political background to Law 180, the Mayor, who represents the local authority on both a political and administrative level, is the supervisor of compulsory health treatment and "the problem of safeguarding society from illness and infirmity becomes a political responsibility" (Basaglia, 1980). In all three countries, psychiatrists only have the role of expert witnesses. Mental health legislation is derived as an exemption from basic human rights that are guaranteed by written constitutions. These guarantees can only be annulled by specific laws brought into action by a judge.

In contrast, the UK has a "complex legislative system" (Curran & Harding, 1978) without a normative setting of laws and sublaws and without a written constitution. Each case of patient detention is considered by psychiatric professionals on its own merits. The mental health tribunal is distinct from the ordinary legal system.

There are also, however, important differences between continental countries. In Germany, dangerousness is a necessary criterion for detention, while in Italy and Spain it is not. This is an important issue dividing 'needs-orientated' from 'rights-orientated' systems. Segal (1989) has analysed the thinking behind the two systems and the repercussions for the admitted populations. In his view, 'needs-orientated' countries are consistent with paternalistic social philosophies prevalent in the welfare states, while countries which emphasise individual rights use the dangerousness criterion as a way to limit compulsory admissions, dealing only with more difficult patients in the face of limited resources.

Conclusions

All EC countries are signatories to the European Convention of Human Rights and the Council of Europe (1985), which guarantee the humane and adequate treatment of patients and their right of appeal. However, the convention provides only a broad definition of "unsoundness of mind" and no criteria for dangerousness or need of treatment. Harmonisation between the different medico-legal positions in Europe seems to be a very difficult task, due to the underlying differences in philosophy, law, legal and medical training in the countries concerned.

Mental health legislation has been in a state of dynamic flux since its beginnings and this is likely to continue. However, it seems to us that consideration of the following questions may help to shape future developments:

(a) Is the compulsory involvement of legally authorised persons in some continental countries too legalistic? Does it damage a patient to be questioned by a judge? Is the Italian model a valid compromise?

(b) Does the Mental Health Act of England and Wales provide legal protection and certainty about the patient's position? Is there too much power in the hands of responsible medical officers and hospital administrators in the UK (Wood, 1993)?

(c) Does the emphasis on the dangerousness criterion favour repeated admissions of patients who cannot be helped by this measure, which serves merely to protect society for a limited time?

(d) Is the UK emphasis on the need for treatment criterion too restrictive and ungracious? Does the Mental Health Act 1983 do justice to patients on the borderline between mental illness and social impairment?

References

BASAGLIA, F. (1980) Problems of law and psychiatry: the Italian experience. *International Journal of Law & Psychiatry*, **3**, 17–37.

COUNCIL OF EUROPE (1985) *Article 5 of the European Convention of Human Rights*. Strasbourg: Council of Europe.

CURRAN, W. J. & HARDING, T. W. (1978) *The Law & Mental Health: Harmonizing Objectives*. Geneva: WHO.

DAVID, R. & JAUFFRET SPINOSI, C. (1988) *Les Grands Systemes de Droit Contemporains* (9th edn). Paris: Dalloz.

DEPARTMENT OF HEALTH AND SOCIAL SECURITY (1984) *The Mental Health Act 1983*. London: HMSO.

EBERHARD, G. A. (ed.) (1980) *Hilfen und Schutzmasnahmen bei psychischen Krankheiten in Nordrhein-Westfalen* (2nd edn). Köln: Deutscher Gemeindeverlag.

HESSE, K. (1984) *Grundzuge des Verfassungsrechts der Bundesrepublik Deutschland* (14th edn). Heidelberg: CF Müller, Juristischer Verlag.

MARSCHNER, R. (1986) Plädoyer für die Abschaffung der zivilrechtlichen Unterbringung. *Recht und Psychiatrie*, **2**, 47–52.

ORTEGA-MONASTERIO, L. (1991) Psiquitria juridica y forense. In *Introduction a la psicopatologia y psiquiatria*. Barcelona: Masson-Salvat.

PIZZI, A. (1978) *Malattie Mentali e Trattamenti Sanitari*. Commento alla legge 13/5/78, no. 180, Giuffre editore, Milan.

ROSE, N. (1986) Law, rights and psychiatry. In *The Power of Psychiatry* (eds P. Miller & N. Rose). Oxford: Polity Press, Blackwell.

SCULL, A. (1984) The theory and practice of civil commitment. *Michigan Law Review*, **82**, 793–809.

SEGAL, S. P. (1989) Civil commitment standards and patient mix in England & Wales, Italy and United States. *American Journal of Psychiatry*, **146**, 187–193.

SMITH, R. (1991) Legal frameworks for psychiatry. In *150 Years of British Psychiatry, 1841–1991*. London: Gaskell.

SOOTHILL, K. (1990) Compulsory admissions to mental hospitals: a replication study. *International Journal of Law and Psychiatry*, **13**, 179–90.

———, HARDING, T. W., ADSERBALLE, H., *et al* (1981) Compulsory admissions to mental hospitals in six countries. *International Journal of Law and Psychiatry*, **4**, 327–344.

WOOD, J. (1993) Reform of the Mental Health Act 1983: an effective tribunal. *British Journal of Psychiatry*, **162**, 14–22.

14 'Psychosomatic medicine' in the general hospital

THOMAS HERZOG, FRANCIS CREED,
FRITS J. HUYSE, ULRIK F. MALT,
ANTONIO LOBO, BARBARA STEIN
and the EUROPEAN CONSULTATION –
LIAISON WORKGROUP

Close professional collaboration between groups from different countries tends to stress the similarities. Whichever language is used as the lingua franca of the day sets the frame of reference. Because of the different use of the words in different countries, the terms 'psychiatry' and 'psychosomatics' may be easily misunderstood when used across boundaries of culture and language. In Germany, a unique system of psychosocial care delivery has developed over the past hundred years which is characterised by two main traditions and approaches: that of general psychiatry, and that of psychosomatics and psychotherapy. Preliminary data from an ongoing collaborative study illustrate the difference that specialised psychosomatics may make in the general hospital.

'Psychosomatics'

To understand the scope and meaning of the term in the German context, we need to consider its history. Figure 14.1 gives a schematic overview. We will focus on the two most important aspects: (a) the special origins of psychosomatics; and (b) the concept of a 'critical medicine' in the aftermath of the Nazi horrors.

Historical and cultural background

Psychosomatics stems from two traditions *outside* psychiatry: (a) internists striving towards more holistic care with a 'psychosomatic' approach to their patients; and (b) psychoanalysts dealing with hysteria (Freud & Breuer, 1985), later applying psychodynamic thinking to patients with other physical complaints and eventually also to physical illness in general. Both traditions

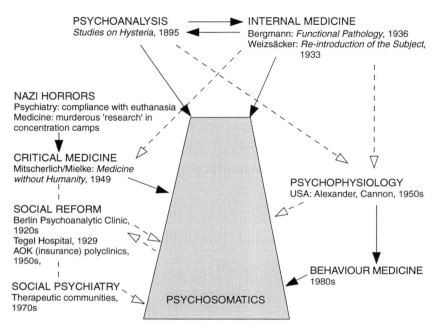

Fig. 14.1. Development of psychosomatics in Germany: theoretical and social influences

reach back at least as far as the 1920s. Even then they were concerned with a critical outlook on conventional medicine. The internist Bergmann reverted to the traditional idea that impaired function followed from structural organic lesions since they could also produce disturbed function. The neurologist and physiologist Weizsäcker wrote about the necessity to "re-introduce the subject, the individual, into medicine", meaning that many symptoms and illnesses could only be adequately understood and treated if taken in the context of an individual biography and living situation (Henningsen, 1990). Psychoanalysis provided such a framework with the concept of a psychical 'apparatus'. At the same time, it was concerned with the psychological and living situation of the working class and with social reform in general, which resulted, for example, in the first psychoanalytic out-patient clinic in Berlin (Simmel, 1930).

'Critical medicine'

This critical impetus gained enormous momentum through the experiences of Nazi fascism. Much of the idiosyncratic development of German psychosomatics came after the Second World War, including the long neglected psychophysiology, which can only be understood by taking into account the attempts to deal with the Nazi experience. A key to this is the report on the Nuremberg trials, *Medicine without Humanity* (Mitscherlich & Mielke, 1949). Psychiatry had failed by making itself accomplice to the Nazi euthanasia programmes, forsaking its own patients. Scientific medicine had failed by perverting the detached objective attitude of the scientist when concentration camp inmates were tortured to death in the name of medical ''experimentation''. The fact that medicine and psychiatry had so easily lent themselves to these perversions of objectifying, classifying and ''statistical'' science, and that the medical establishment reacted with some hostility to Mitscherlich & Mielke's report, was taken as further proof that radical changes were needed throughout medicine, and that objectification was to be viewed sceptically. From this has resulted a continuing interest in social reform. The recruitment of doctors who were dissatisfied with traditional medicine or psychiatry, and who were open to disciplines like psychology or sociology, is another consequence. Whereas psychopathology was often shunned, and psychiatric diagnoses were often avoided in order not to ''stigmatise'' and ''deindividualise'' the patient, social psychiatric developments could be more easily assimilated. For example, all psychosomatic/psychotherapeutic in-patient treatment is indebted to the therapeutic community (Herzog, 1991*a*).

Present state of psychosomatics

Since the early 1980s, cognitive–behavioural and systemic approaches, based in some hospitals and in most psychology departments, have become increasingly important. Simultaneously, empirical research of psychotherapy and of the evaluation of different therapies and settings has soared. Pragmatic approaches, trying to combine or even integrate whatever seemed to fit best with the needs of a particular patient, steadily gained ground. At present, the more recent cognitive–behavioural 'schools' tend to be more orthodox and one-sided than the older psychodynamic ones. However, apart from some competition for funding and prestige, these two major approaches mostly cross-fertilise each other, both theoretically and in the practice of care-delivery.

It is important to take account of some structural peculiarities. The boom in in-patient psychotherapy that led to the creation of almost 8000 in-patient treatment places has much to do with other special features of the German system of health care delivery and financing (Herzog, 1991*a*). *Out-patient therapy* in psychosomatics basically means psychotherapy. This is influenced by two special aspects of the German system of obligatory health insurance: (a) out-patient services are strictly separated from in-patient services; and (b) since 1967 psychotherapy has been established as a medical treatment to which everyone in need is entitled. On application by the patient, up to 300 psychotherapy sessions will be paid for, provided the treatment plan is approved by an independent expert.

Specialist and general training in psychosomatics received a boost through the creation of a new medical speciality, the 'Arzt für psychotherapeutische Medizin', requiring five years of full-time training focusing on psychological interventions in the medical context. Apart from this, every doctor, whether general practitioner or specialist, can obtain psychotherapy training (three years part-time) and then do formal psychotherapy in addition to his other work. The trainee can emphasise either psychodynamic or cognitive–behavioural approaches in his training and future practice. This training, increasingly provided by departments of psychotherapy and psychosomatics, is an important means to spread the *psychosomatic* approach, which aims to build a bridge between the various clinical specialities, overcoming the body and mind dichotomy by stressing the interactions between biological, psychological and social factors in every patient (Herzog, 1991*b*). The training of every doctor in integrating this approach into everyday practice (theory, case discussions, psychosocial skills) is greatly helped by the recent introduction of a qualification in 'psychosomatic basic care', and the possibility to budget for it in all out-patient medicine. Psychosomatics contributes much of the necessary material and supervision.

Psychosocial care for in-patients in Germany

Psychosocial care delivery to the general hospital in-patient calls for cooperation, usually in the form of consultation–liaison (CL) work (Mayou *et al*, 1991). There are two general stances in CL work, the relative merits of which are much debated, so far with little empirical research into what is actually done and whether it affects patients and consultee differently. These two approaches are *strict integration* and *integration by cooperation* (Herzog, 1991*b*). Those who hold a strictly integrative view of the psychosomatic approach tend to oppose psychosomatics as a distinct speciality, because every doctor should fully integrate psychosocial aspects and should need cooperation only in cases of the core psychiatric illnesses. Consultation requests for other problems are considered to be due to insufficient training or interest. Cooperation – if it needs to be practised at all – should be staff-oriented as opposed to patient-oriented and it should be more intensive, at least in the form of a *liaison* service, in order to fulfil its training function towards integration of all relevant aspects within one person/team.

On the other hand, integration by cooperation allows for the limitations of the individual, who may find it impossible or even undesirable to be both an expert physician and an expert in psychological medicine. Psychological diagnosis and treatment is seen as a skill that requires considerable competence and experience when applied to patients with physical complaints, and requires full specialist training and identity. This view accepts the traditional *consultation* as one important way to cooperate. Both positions agree that liaison servies can increase the rate of timely and appropriate referrals, thereby improving diagnosis and treatment of psychological disorder.

Psychiatric and psychosomatic CL services

Psychiatrists, depending on where they work, see all types of patients, but focus mostly on those with organic brain syndromes including deliria, substance abuse and severe schizophreniform and affective disorders (i.e. those disorders with a fairly clear-cut biological basis and with some susceptibility to biological treatments). From 1992 on, some basic psychotherapeutic skills will form part of every psychiatrist's training. Psychosomatics deals with the whole range of non-psychotic and non-organic psychological disorders, with a special emphasis on those presenting with some kind of physical complaint and on issues of coping and compliance. Patients with functional, neurotic and personality disorders make up the largest part of their clientele. Psychotherapy is the main treatment in psychosomatics and is provided in all kinds of settings and using all kinds of theoretical frameworks.

Availability of CL services

Of the 1800 general hospitals in what used to be West Germany, only about 180 have in-hospital mental health services available. The remainder are served haphazardly by external psychiatrists, always in addition to their normal full work load. The existing in-hospital CL services are provided by psychosomatics in about 20% of cases, and by psychiatry in about 95%, which means that psychosomatic departments are rarely the sole providers of psychological medicine, whereas psychiatric ones usually have to cover the whole range of problems. A recent survey (Herzog & Hartmann, 1990) showed that most of the general hospital psychiatric departments have some specialised competence in psychotherapy and psychosomatics, just as the psychosomatic departments usually have fully trained psychiatrists on their CL staff.

Evidence for differences between CL services

The collaborative study on consultation–liaison psychiatry and psychosomatics in the general hospital conducted by the European Consultation Liaison Workgroup (ECLW) provides a unique opportunity for comparing different CL services. To illustrate the possible impact of psychosomatics, data from eight UK and 11 German (five psychiatric and

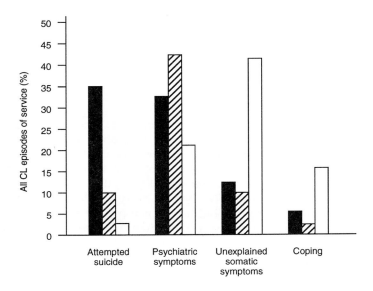

Fig. 14.2. Primary reason for referral to psychiatric and psychosomatic CL services. ■, *UK psychiatric;* ▨, *German psychiatric;* ☐, *German psychosomatic*

six psychosomatic) CL services were collected from consecutive referrals, using reliable and comprehensive diagnostics (ICD–10) and descriptions of case episodes (Huyse, 1990; Huyse *et al*, 1993; Herzog *et al*, 1994). Data entry and analysis are still under way, but on the basis of over 3000 CL episodes (about 1000 from each type of service), some trends emerge.

Patients seen by the different services

The primary reason for referral (Fig. 14.2) reflects the expectations of the consultees concerning the CL services and their competence. The strikingly higher proportion of attempted suicides in the UK is probably explained by epidemiological, legal and health service peculiarities. Unexplained physical symptoms and problems coping with physical illness account for more than half the patients referred to psychosomatics, as opposed to less than a quarter in both psychiatric samples.

Assuming similar base rates of medical diagnoses among admissions to UK and German general hospitals, as well as sufficient diagnostic reliability, safeguarded by ECLW training, it seems that patients with certain psychiatric diagnoses (neurotic, stress-related and adjustment disorders, behavioural syndromes associated with physiological disturbances and physical factors) are grossly underrepresented where psychosomatic CL services or a psychosomatic orientation of a CL service are lacking

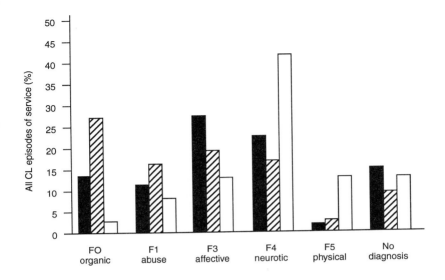

Fig. 14.3. Psychiatric diagnoses (ICD–10) from psychiatric and psychosomatic CL services. ■, *UK psychiatric;* ▨ , *German psychiatric;* □ , *German psychosomatic*

(Fig. 14.3). The German consultees already have clear ideas of who can do what. The somewhat intermediate position of the UK sample probably reflects the lack of specialisation.

Approaches to the psychosomatic patient

In order to compare approaches used by the different types of service towards patients with non-organic psychiatric disorder, we pragmatically defined a patient as 'psychosomatic' if he/she presents with physical symptoms or signs caused or influenced by psychological factors or with psychological reactions to illness complicating the latter. From the different CL services, a subsample of 476 psychosomatic patients matched for age, sex and clinical features was drawn, about 50 % from the German psychosomatic CL services and about 25 % each from the German and UK psychiatric CL services.

Psychiatrists generally spend less than half the time on these patients that psychosomatic practitioners do, independent of manpower, probably because psychosomatic consultants assess indications for out-patient psychotherapy and try to motivate patients for it, sometimes with remarkable compliance rates (Jordan *et al*, 1989). The most clear-cut differences concern the relative importance of biological interventions. There is a clear tendency for psychosomatic services to decrease medical treatments, in keeping with their tradition of 'critical medicine'. This specifically concerns the issue of medication. For the same type of patient and problem, psychiatric consultants prescribe medication in up to 60% of cases, but psychosomaticists in less than 5%, indicating that theoretical orientation has a greater influence on what is done and suggested than diagnosis and other patient-related variables.

Does psychosomatic medicine make a difference?

Firstly, it is different. The historical and institutional background has shaped the psychosomatic approach, which has a strong systemic component, taking a historical perspective and always looking for the meaning of the symptom in the context of an individual biography. In this sense, the idiosyncratic development of psychosomatic medicine in Germany is a symptom of the country's peculiar history.

Secondly, it does make a difference. Psychosomatic patients, according to the rather wide definition proposed, seem grossly underrepresented in UK CL services. It may be that UK physicians and surgeons are less aware of the problems of this group of patients, or that they are less confident that the consultant can help. Perhaps this has also to do with a lack of interest from the consultants themselves, or psychiatry as a discipline, in reaching out to other fields and educating other doctors. Notwithstanding the ubiquitous difficulties in cooperating with mental health and medical services, it seems that in the German hospitals the consultees have been educated well enough to recognise the complementarity of psychiatric and psychosomatic services and make fairly specific referrals. Whether psychosomatics makes a difference in terms of outcomes remains to be seen. The methodological problems in CL research sometimes seem overwhelming. Also, the question of outcomes needs to be seen in perspective. Whether one treats a psychosomatic patient with pills or with some form of a talking cure or with both is not just a matter of cost-effectiveness that can be decided without regard to culture and circumstance. Cost-effectiveness issues must take account of the values which all parties involved – the patient and his family, the consultees and consultants, society, and so on – place on certain decisions and procedures. The data do seem to indicate that, without a psychosomatic orientation, the patients we defined as psychosomatic are often neglected, underrecognised and possibly not treated adequately. This also has economic implications; according to our preliminary data they are often frequent users of medical services and show a profile of chronic but unrecognised psychosocial impairment.

The whole field could greatly benefit from taking more account of the psychotherapists and their accumulated clinical wisdom, and of empirical psychotherapy research. At least in principle, this seems to be more advanced where specialised psychosomatics are available.

References

FREUD, S. & BREUER, J. (orig. 1895) Studies on hysteria. *The Standard Edition of the Complete Psychological Works of Sigmund Freud, vol. 2*, 1953–1974. London: Hogarth.

HENNINGSEN, P. (1990) *Was "leistet" die Psychosomatische Medizin im Unterschied zur naturwissenschaftlichen Medizin? Eine Literaturstudie (1965–1989)*. Heidelberg: Protestant Institute for Interdisciplinary Research.

HERZOG, T. (1991*a*) Psychosomatic liaison services. In *The European Handbook of Psychiatry and Mental Health* (ed. A. Seva), 1447–1455. Barcelona: Anthropos.

—— (1991*b*) Inpatient treatment with patients with severe psychosomatic and neurotic disorders – a German perspective. *British Journal of Psychotherapy*, **8**, 189–198.

—— & HARTMANN, A. (1990) Psychiatrische, psychosomatische und medizinpsychologische Konsiliar- und Liaisontätigkeit in der Bundesrepublik Deutschland. Ergebnisse einer Umfrage. *Nervenarzt*, **61**, 281–293.

——, STEIN, B., FICKER, F., *et al* (1994) Konsiliar/Liaison-Psychiatrie und Psychosomatik in Deutschland und die deutsche Verbundstudie der ECLW. In *150 Jahre Psychiatrie* (eds U. H. Peters, M. Schifferdecker & A. Krahl). Köln: Martini Verlag.

HUYSE, F. J. (1990) Consultation–liaison psychiatry. Does it help to get organized? *General Hospital Psychiatry*, **13**, 183–187.

——, HERZOG, T., MALT, U. F., *et al* (1993) The effectiveness of mental health service delivery in the general hospital. In *Health Services Research* (eds G. N. Fracchia & M. Theofilatou), pp. 227–242. Amsterdam: IOS Press.

JORDAN, J., SAPPER, H., SCHIMKE, H., *et al* (1989) Zur Wirksamkeit des patientenzentrierten psychosomatischen Konsiliardienstes. *Psychotherapie, Psychosomatik, Medizinische Psychologie*, **39**, 127–134.

MAYOU, R., HUYSE, F. J. & ECLW (1991) Consultation–liaison psychiatry in western Europe. *General Hospital Psychiatry*, **13**, 188–209.

MITSCHERLICH, A. & MIELKE, F. (orig. 1949) *Medizin ohne Menschlichkeit. Dokumente des Nürnberger Ärzteprozesses*. Frankfurt: Suhrkamp (1984).

SIMMEL, E. (1930) Zur Geschichte und sozialen Bedeutung des Berliner Psychoanalytischen Institutes. In *Zehn Jahre Berliner Psychoanalytisches Institut* (ed. Deutsche Psychoanalytische Gesellschaft). Wien: Internationaler Psychoanalytischer Verlag.

15 Day treatment and community care in the Netherlands

DURK WIERSMA, ROBERT GIEL and HERMAN KLUITER

In the Netherlands, the number of mental hospital beds has, since the 1970s, remained stable at 1.5 per 1000 of the population. This is remarkable because the same number has been created for psychogeriatric patients, and an even greater number for the mentally retarded. Both categories of patients, in the meantime, have been disappearing from the mental hospitals. Although mental health care policy is focusing on a reduction of hospitalisation, and on community care and sheltered accommodation, it appears that a true reduction in the number of beds is difficult to achieve.

According to a World Health Organization (WHO) report (WHO, 1987), day treatment, community care and continuity of care are rare in Europe for patients with major psychiatric disorders. There was great pressure from the patient movement to stop renovation of mental hospitals, and to create new services (van der Poel *et al*, 1985), but research supporting such alternatives was rare in the Netherlands. For example, Jenner (1984) developed "admission preventing strategies" and claimed their effectiveness from the decreasing admission rates in the area where he practised, compared with national averages. A controlled study of chronic schizophrenics (Asselbergs, 1989; Vlaminck, 1989) showed that intensive community care and individual guidance could reduce the number of readmissions and relapses. Haveman *et al* (1986), investigating the possibility of transfer of the long-stay population into the community, established that in the opinion of hospital staff about one in three long stay patients (more than two years in hospital) could be relocated, if adequate facilities were available to them. However, it was left open how much time this would require. Giel (1986) concluded that in spite of expanded extramural care the number of in-patients over a period of five years (1976–1981) had remained at about 4 per 1000 of the population. He was quite sceptical about the possibilities of community-based care for the chronically mentally ill, and he warned against a great reduction in mental hospital beds.

The number of 'new' long-stay patients with a mean stay of 2–5 years has indeed been increasing from 13.7% of the total mental hospital population in 1986, to 15.2% in 1990 (Nationaal Ziekenhuis instituut (NZi), 1992), indicating that various forms of day treatment, out-patient and community care are not sufficiently effective to prevent institutionalisation.

Day treatment

In the Netherlands, day treatment or partial hospitalisation dates back to 1961, and has increased in 30 years to 90 institutions (Jacobs & Bijl, 1992), each with an average of 32 places. In 1990 more than 8000 patients were accepted for treatment. The number of patients per place is 1.7. It is one of the fastest growing types of institution. Compared with 1982, the number of patients in treatment has increased by 174%, annual enrolment by 73%, and the number of patients per place by 42%.

According to Schene *et al* (1986), who conducted a nationwide survey, four categories of day treatment can be distinguished: (a) as an alternative to full-time hospitalisation, (b) as a continuation of full-time hospitalisation, (c) as an extension of out-patient or ambulatory treatment, (d) as day care or rehabilitation for chronic patients. Most patients were referred to these services because they offer extra out-patient treatment (40%), or as a continuation of in-patient treatment (30%). Day care for chronic patients accounted for 14%. Only 9% of the patients used it as an alternative to full-time hospitalisation.

Staffing, patient population, contraindications, treatment programme and duration of treatment varied depending on the intentions of the service (Schene *et al*, 1986). For example, patients referred to day treatment as an extension of ambulatory care tended to be younger and more highly educated, with a predominance of neurotic, personality or depressive disorders. Selection is strict, and treatment is intensive and protracted, with a psychotherapeutic orientation. Facilities are often located at some distance from the main psychiatric institutions, in contrast to day treatment as a continuation of full-time hospitalisation; this is usually situated close to a mental hospital. A large proportion of its patients attend the service for part of the week only. Patients tend to be older and less educated. They suffer more often from psychoses, and they are usually referred by the hospital. Treatment is much less psychotherapeutically oriented.

Day treatment used as an alternative to inpatient treatment was rare. In 1986, 9% or some 270 patients annually used such a facility because "it is anticipated that they will otherwise have to be hospitalised within a week" (Schene *et al*, 1988). This kind of day treatment mostly takes place in the mental hospital, and staff/patient ratios are relatively high.

In summary, day treatment is currently still a rather limited treatment modality in terms of places and staff. Only 2.4% of the mental health care budget is assigned to this type of treatment (Jacobs & Bijl, 1992).

Community care

Since 1980, the development of the RIAGGs, the Regional Institutes for Ambulatory Care, is a unique feature of out-patient and ambulatory care in the Netherlands. The RIAGGs provide mental health promotion, treatment and care, including all kinds of psychotherapy and aftercare, to all children, adults and elderly in their catchment areas. The 60 RIAGGs in the Netherlands form the main gateway to and from intramural psychiatric care. Numbers of staff have grown by more than 50% since 1980, to 4700 in 1990 (Jacobs & Bijl, 1992). Community psychiatric nurses, social workers, psychologists and psychotherapists are most numerous; only 7% are psychiatrists. The number of enrolled and treated patients increased from 19.3 per 1000 inhabitants in 1987, to 24.8 in 1990. Towards the end of 1990, about 228 900 patients were in active treatment, that is, 15.4 per 1000 of the population. Two-thirds of all patients are between 20 and 65 years old, 15% are younger and 18% are older.

The RIAGGs operate round-the-clock for crisis intervention and the prevention of admission: 3.6% of all face-to-face contacts are in this type of intervention (NVAGG, 1991). From its history and ideology, the RIAGG can be considered the natural 'opponent' of the mental hospital. National policy, therefore, has focused on transferring part of the hospital budget to the RIAGGs, although not with a great deal of success. Only 13.2% of the mental health care budget is spent on ambulatory and community care (Jacobs & Bijl, 1992), while over the last five years the average annual increase of the budget has been larger for mental hospitals than for community services: 4.8% versus 3.6%.

Research

In order to emphasise national policy on the substitution of in-patient care, two investigations were started in the mid-1980s directed at the feasibility of day treatment as an alternative.

One study, conducted by the Department of Social Psychiatry of the University of Groningen, took place in a modern 500-bed mental hospital in a semi-rural area in northern Holland (see Wiersma *et al*, 1991, 1994; Kluiter *et al*, 1992; Rüphan *et al*, 1992; Nienhuis *et al*, 1994). The other study was located in the psychiatric department of the University Hospital in Utrecht, the fourth largest city in the Netherlands; this psychiatric department had closed and open wards. The research was conducted by the Department of Psychiatry of the University of Utrecht (see Poelijoe, 1992; Schene, 1992). Both studies were randomised controlled trials. The Groningen study hoped to generalise to the patient population of mental hospitals, and the Utrecht study aimed at generalising to the patient population admitted to the open wards of psychiatric departments of general hospitals.

The control treatment in both studies comprised standard clinical care in a modern mental hospital, with medication, regular contacts with a psychiatrist, occupational therapy, and in indicated cases, individual, group, behavioural, creative or psychomotor therapy. Aftercare was mainly provided by the RIAGG or the general practitioner.

The experimental condition took place in the same hospital and consisted of new forms of day treatment. In both settings, a separate day hospital was created, closely connected with the clinical units. In the Groningen study, day treatment was integrated with ambulatory and domiciliary care provided by the RIAGG, aiming at ruling out total hospitalisation and creating more continuity and flexibility of care. This day centre had a capacity of 8–10 patients, to whom a specially conceived multidisciplinary programme was offered. Day treatment could also take place in a regular clinical unit, where the patient participated in the usual day programme, while spending the night at home. Day treatment could be interrupted for one or more nights (''a bed on prescription''). In case of problems, a special telephone line was available to patients 24 hours a day. Aftercare was initiated by the RIAGG upon admission, and not after discharge as in the control condition.

The Utrecht study had no such link with the ambulatory service. Day treatment took place in a new day hospital of 24 places, offering a similar programme as in the in-patient units. Three parallel programmes were available to a heterogeneous patient populations. The day hospital had two community psychiatric nurses on its staff. It also had an overnight guestroom, a bed on the open in-patient unit, and a telephone service.

Both studies were longitudinal, for two years and six months after discharge respectively. Interviews were held with the patient and his/her relatives at various points in time. Both studies used to a large extent the same standardised instruments with respect to patient's symptoms (PSE; Wing *et al*, 1974) and social disabilities (GSDS; Wiersma *et al*, 1988). The burden on the family and the satisfaction with care were measured on several occasions. All treatment was registered in detail during follow-up.

Issues of evaluation

Evaluation of the ''substitution'' approach focused on four issues (Wiersma & Giel, 1991):

(a) *feasibility*: to what extent is this kind of day treatment feasible for the population of patients being admitted to a mental hospital, or to a psychiatric department of a general hospital?

(b) *substitution*: how many beds can actually be substituted by day places?

(c) *prevention*: to what extent does day treatment alter the course of the illness, psychosocial functioning of the patient and his dependency on mental health care?

(d) *functional coherence*: to what extent are hospital, out-patient and community services better integrated than before, with more continuity and flexibility of care?

Feasibility

In the Groningen study (Kluiter *et al*, 1992), characterised by the intention-to-treat, an average of four or more nights per week at home was considered feasible. It appeared that according to this criterion, 39% of the patient population could be placed in day treatment. Although no absolute contraindications were found, its feasibility was to a certain degree dependent on the patient not being physically ill, on having been admitted for symptoms of depression, and on being admitted for the first time. Day treatment was equally successful in the case of readmission during follow-up; 42% of the patients who had to be readmitted after the index admission could be treated in a day setting. This is remarkable because of the greater number of chronic and alcohol-addicted patients among them.

In the Utrecht study the feasibility criterion depended on the ability of the patient to complete at least one full week of day treatment. According to this criterion, about 33% of the admitted population could successfully be placed in day treatment. Again, no clear contraindications could be established. Feasibility in both studies was not related to higher doses of pharmaceuticals.

Substitution

In both studies, hospital beds have been replaced by an equal number of places in a day treatment setting, while retaining the functions of intensive treatment and round-the-clock care for acute disturbed patients. We concluded that the new day treatment had indeed achieved its goal. Patients were comparable to local and national patient populations. There was no evidence according to case register data in the Groningen study (Giel & ten Horn, 1982) that patterns of referral and care had changed due to the experiment. Neither were new categories of patients attracted, or old ones kept away or referred to other hospitals.

Day patients tended to use the services more than controls. In both studies, day treatment took more time than the standard in-patient treatment, in particular in the Utrecht study (50% more). Ambulatory and out-patient care for day patients, particularly in the Groningen study, was more frequent; this was expected because of the involvement of the RIAGG.

These findings mean that about 2900 mental hospital beds could be replaced by day places. This is 33% of the estimated 9000 beds in mental hospitals used for treatment up to two years (with about 30 000 admissions annually). For the 2100 beds in psychiatric departments of general hospitals (short stay beds, with 17 000 admissions annually), this would result in a reduction of 700 beds.

Prevention

Prevention refers to the reduction or avoidance of chronicity and disablement. Compared with standard clinical care, day treatment was equally successful in reducing psychopathology. At one and two years follow-up, patients did not differ with respect to psychiatric symptoms, impairment of psychological functions, course of the illness, and average duration of episodes. The same applied to the improvement of social role functioning in the family, social relationships, or occupational role. Day patients in the Groningen study performed significantly better concerning self-care, and they had shorter periods of problems with self-care and in the family.

Day treatment did not alter the rate of readmissions: 40% in the Groningen study during follow-up of two years, and 25% within six months of discharge in the Utrecht study. This did not result in a greater burden on the family. Day patients were inclined to resume their tasks in the household earlier and more easily (particularly in the Groningen study; cf. Fenton *et al*, 1979).

Functional coherence

Functional coherence of mental health care is an important objective of health planners and managers. It strengthens efficiency and effectiveness, and is fundamental to establishing continuity, particularly for a population of chronic patients. In the Groningen study, the new day treatment brought together hospital and RIAGG staff for planning and coordination of the treatment of each patient, at the time of his first screening, during admission, and at discharge. The RIAGG staff were members of the day hospital team and carried full responsibility for some patients, even during admission. Ambulatory and community care were intensified during the episode of day treatment and during follow-up.

Conclusions

Day treatment is feasible for about three to four out of every ten patients in need of admission, either to a mental hospital or to a psychiatric department of a general hospital (Wiersma & Schene, 1992). The findings of Zwerling & Wilder (1964) in New York, and of Creed *et al* (1990, 1991) in the UK are in line with ours. There are no absolute contraindications (e.g. psychosis, the threat of suicide, or compulsory admission). Feasibility does not depend on more medication and did not cause extra burden to the family. The effects on the course of psychopathology and on social functioning are equivalent to standard clinical care.

We established that the direct costs of illness in terms of the number of days in (day) hospital and of ambulatory and community contacts did not show great differences between the two conditions. Time spent by staff with patients was roughly the same in both treatment settings. Extra costs for travelling or for community care were marginal compared with the total treatment costs, in which hospital costs prevailed. The extra costs to the RIAGG were partly compensated for by a reorientation of its staff towards serving the more chronically mentally ill (instead of mainly helping patients with psychosocial problems) and partly by increased efficiency.

For a cost–benefit analysis (cf. Drummond *et al*, 1987; Glass & Goldberg, 1977), the benefit has to be emphasised of patients spending less time in secluded wards and remaining longer "in the least restrictive environment possible", being more satisfied with their care, and doing better in the long term concerning self-care and the skills of daily life. Patients did not fare better with respect to recurrences of psychopathology or their dependency on care. Particularly for chronic patients, service utilisation had intensified continuity and flexibility of care. This resulted in greater compliance (i.e. fewer discharges against medical advice, same readmission rate, longer duration of treatment episodes), which has to be considered a favourable outcome, and not a failure or a new route to institutionalisation (Tantam & McGrath, 1989).

This 'substitution' model should not be seen as a single new service, but as a differentiation of clinical care in a new form of day treatment (e.g. on a ward, or in a day hospital), with close links with ambulatory and extramural care. 'Admission to a bed' has been transformed into a flexible and open arrangement. An important factor is the recognition of joint responsibility of the various components in the service network for chronic patients from the catchment area. We expect growth of day treatment in several directions, not just for patients with neurotic and personality problems rarely requiring full-time hospitalisation, or for patients with serious and chronic psychiatric problems after a period of in-patient treatment, but also for patients in need of acute full-time admission. Recent developments in policy (e.g. abandonment of central planning, and the rigid sectorisation of mental health care) provide new opportunities for substitution and collaboration. Home care or treatment together with crisis and mobile treatment teams and more emphasis on rehabilitation (Stein & Test, 1980; Hoult, 1990) will hopefully follow.

References

ASSELBERGS, L. (1989) Sociaal beperkt (Socially disabled). An empirical study into the social functioning of schizophrenic patients in the Psychosis Prevention Project in Rotterdam. Thesis, University of Utrecht.

CREED, F., BLACK, D., ANTHONY, P., et al (1990) Randomised controlled trial comparing day and in-patient psychiatric treatment. *British Medical Journal*, **300**, 1033–1037.

——, ——, ——, et al (1991) Randomised controlled trial of day patients and in-patient psychiatric treatment. II: Comparison of two hospitals. *British Journal of Psychiatry*, **158**, 183–189.

DRUMMOND, M. F., STODDART, F. L. & TORRANCE, G. W. (1987) *Methods for the Economic Evaluation of Health Care Programmes*. Oxford: Oxford University Press.

FENTON, F. R., TESSIER, L. & STRUENING, E. L. (1979) A comparative trial of home and hospital care. One year follow up. *Archives of General Psychiatry*, **36**, 1073–1079.

GIEL, R. (1986) Care of chronic mental patients in the Netherlands. *Social Psychiatry*, **21**, 25–32.

—— & TEN HORN, G. H. M. M. (1982) Patterns of mental health care in a Dutch register area. *Social Psychiatry*, **17**, 117–123.

GLASS, N. J. & GOLDBERG, D. (1977) Cost benefit analysis and the evaluation of psychiatric services. *Psychological Medicine*, **7**, 701–717.

HAVEMAN, M. J., POELIJOE, N. W. & TAN, E. S. (1986) *Vervangende Zorg voor Lang Opgenomen Patienten in Psychiatrische Ziekenhuizen: Verslag van een Landelijk Substitutieonderzoek*. Maastricht: University of Limburg.

HOULT, J. (1990) Dissemination in New South Wales of the Madison model. In *Mental Health Care Delivery. Innovations, Impediments and Implementation* (eds I. M. Marks & R. A. Scott). Cambridge: Cambridge University Press.

JACOBS, C. M. V. W. & BIJL, R. V. (1992) *GGZ in Getallen 1992*. Utrecht: National centrum Geestelijke volksge-zondheid.

JENNER, J. A. (1984) *Opnamevoorkomende Strategieën in de Praktijk van de Sociale Psychiatrie*. Thesis, Erasmus University, Rotterdam.

KLUITER, H., GIEL, R., NIENHUIS, F. J., et al (1992) Predicting feasibility of day-treatment for unselected patients in need of admission: results from a randomized trial. *American Journal of Psychiatry*, **149**, 1199–1205.

NATIONAAL ZIEKENHUIS INSTITUUT (1992) *Psychiatrische Ziekenhuizen in Cijfers*. Utrecht: Nationaal Ziekenhuis instituut.

NIENHUIS, F. J., GIEL, R., KLUITER, H., et al (1994) Efficacy of psychiatric day treatment. Course and outcome of psychiatric disorders in a randomized trial. *European Archives of Psychiatry and Neurological Sciences*, in press.

NVAGG (1991) *RIAGGs in Cijfers 1989*. Utrecht: NVAGG.

POELIJOE, N. W. (1992) *Opnamevervangende Dagbehandeling op Open Psychiatrische Afdelingen van Algemene Ziekenhuizen*. Thesis, University of Utrecht.

RÜPHAN, M., GIEL, R., KLUITER, H., et al (1992) *Social Role Functioning as a Separate Dimension of Caseness: a Study of Outcome of Day Treatment*. Department of Social Psychiatry, University of Groningen.

SCHENE, A. H. (1992) *Psychiatrische Dagbehandeling en 24-uurs Behandeling: een Vergelijkend Onderzoek*. Thesis, University of Utrecht.

——, VAN LIESHOUT, P. & MASTBOOM, J. (1986) Development and current status of partial hospitalization in the Netherlands. *International Journal of Partial Hospitalization*, **3**, 237–246.

——, —— & —— (1988) Different types of partial hospitalization programs: results of a nationwide survey in the Netherlands. *Acta Psychiatrica Scandinavica*, **78**, 515–522.

STEIN, L. I. & TEST, M. A. (1980) Alternative to mental hospital treatment. Conceptual model, treatment program and clinical evaluation. *Archives of General Psychiatry*, **37**, 392–397.

TANTAM, D. & McGRATH, G. (1989) Psychiatric day hospitals – another route to institutionalisation? *Social Psychiatry and Psychiatric Epidemiology*, **24**, 96–101.

VAN DER POEL, E., ROMME, M., TRIMBOS, K., *et al* (1985) *Het Psychiatrisch Ziekenhuis in Discussie. Verslag van de actie Moratorium Niewbouw APZ-en.*

VLAMINCK, P. (1989) *Ambulante Zorg voor Schizofrene Patienten. Een Pragmatisch Interventieonderzoek.* Thesis, University of Utrecht. Delft: EBURON.

WIERSMA, D., DE JONG, A. & ORMEL, J. (1988) The Groningen Social Disabilities Schedule: Development, relationship with the ICIDH and psychometric properties. *International Journal of Rehabilitative Research*, **11**, 213–224.

—— & GIEL, R. (1991) Evaluation of change in mental health care. In *Evaluation of Comprehensive Care of the Mentally Ill* (eds H. Freeman & J. Henderson). London: Gaskell.

——, KLUITER, H., NIENHUIS, F. J., *et al* (1991) Costs and benefits of day treatment with community care as an alternative to standard hospitalisation for schizophrenic patients: a randomized controlled trial in the Netherlands. *Schizophrenia Bulletin*, **17**, 411–419.

—— & SCHENE, A. H. (eds) (1992) *Opnamevervangende Dagbe-handeling in de Psychiatrie. Resultaten van Onderzoek naar Haalbaarheid en Effecten van Substitutieprojecten in Drenthe en Utrecht.* Utrecht: Nationaal Centrum Geestelijke Volksgezondheid (NcGv).

——, KLUITER, H., NIENHUIS, F. J., *et al* (1994) Costs and benefits of hospital and day treatment with community care of affective and schizophrenic disorders. A randomized trial with a follow up of two years. *British Journal of Psychiatry*, supplement (in press).

WING, J. K., COOPER, J. E. & SARTORIUS, N. (1974) *Measurement and Classification of Psychiatric Symptoms*. Cambridge: Cambridge University Press.

WORLD HEALTH ORGANIZATION (1987) *Mental Health Services in Pilot Study Areas. Report on a European Study.* Copenhagen: WHO Regional Office.

ZWERLING, I. H. & WILDER, J. F. (1964) An evaluation of the application of the day hospital in treatment of acutely disturbed patients. *The Israel Annals of Psychiatry and Related Disciplines*, **2**, 162–185.

16 Teaching and training in child and adolescent psychiatry in Hungary

WILLIAM Ll. PARRY-JONES,
AGNES VETRÓ, ANDREAS WARNKE
and GERHARDT NISSEN

For several years, there have been growing opportunities for scientific and professional exchange between child and adolescent psychiatrists within western Europe but, until recently, this was not the case with those from central and eastern European countries. This chapter describes an innovative, three-year project, ending in August 1993, designed to upgrade and expand the teaching and training of child and adolescent psychiatry in Hungary, involving two university departments in western Europe. This Joint European Project (JEP) was funded by the Trans-European Mobility Scheme for University Studies (TEMPUS) established by the Commission of the European Communities. This scheme was concerned with the development of higher education in central and eastern Europe through cooperation with European Community (EC) universities and the G24 countries (TEMPUS, 1992a). The target group of the scheme included teachers, trainers, students and industrialists in universities and industries in Poland, Hungary, Czechoslovakia, Bulgaria, Romania, Albania, Estonia, Latvia and Lithuania. Of the former Yugoslavia, only Slovenia was included. The TEMPUS programme ran from 1 July 1990 until 30 June 1994. The particular project described in this chapter was one of eight medical sciences projects included in the 11% of successful applications in 1990, and was the only psychiatric project to be accepted (TEMPUS, 1992b).

Child and adolescent psychiatry in Hungary

Child and adolescent psychiatry has been seriously neglected in Hungary and, during the period when the country formed part of the Eastern Bloc, dominated politically and economically by the USSR, its growth did not proceed at the same rate as in western Europe. Although there have been no recent epidemiological studies, clinical experience has suggested rising prevalence of psychiatric disorder in children and adolescents, including, for example, suicidal behaviour, conduct disorder and drug abuse. Suicide rates for all ages in Hungary are already among the highest in the world. Furthermore, at a time of rapid political, economic and social change, accompanying the transformation of communist Hungary into a multi-party republic which began in 1989, there are likely to have been increased levels of psychosocial disturbance. Nevertheless, clinical services remain seriously inadequate and, currently, there are only 74 psychiatrists specialising in child and adolescent psychiatry catering for a total population of 10.5 million. The situation has been compounded by an almost complete lack of undergraduate teaching, postgraduate training and academic input in child and adolescent psychiatry. Of the four Hungarian undergraduate medical universities, at Budapest, Debrecen, Pécs and Szeged, only at the latter has there been any attempt to organise teaching. Not surprisingly, research has been minimal and the recruitment of high calibre staff has been poor.

Since 1968, child and adolescent psychiatry has been recognised as a separate postgraduate medical speciality in Hungary, with independent examinations and training standards set by a committee of the Ministry of Health. The speciality may be entered from general adult psychiatry, neurology or paediatrics. While there are close professional links with general psychiatry, the separate professional identity of child and adolescent psychiatry was strengthened by the establishment, in 1991, of the Hungarian Association of Child Neurology and Child and Adolescent Psychiatry.

Participating centres

Three centres participated in the project, in accordance with the requirement that the consortium should include universities from at least two EC countries. Glasgow University was the contractor, with WLP-J as the project coordinator. AV is in charge of child and adolescent psychiatry in the Department of Pediatrics in Szeged, and AW is the head of the Child and Adolescent Psychiatry Department at Würzburg, Germany, following the retirement of GN, one of the initial applicants. The project was managed by a Project Steering Group, chaired by the coordinator, which met at least twice a year.

Objectives

During initial meetings of the project leaders in 1989–1990, it was evident that rapid development of the speciality in Hungary was needed urgently, and that a substantial increase in the body of adequately trained child and adolescent psychiatrists was required. In order to achieve this, it was decided to set as the general objective the development of undergraduate and postgraduate teaching and training in child and adolescent psychiatry in all Hungarian medical universities. More specifically, the project focused on the upgrading of teaching and training in the small academic unit of child and adolescent psychiatry at Szeged. The assumption was that progress in this centre would generalise to other medical universities and so achieve wider impact. Over three years, the overall plan was to deal, consecutively, with undergraduate curriculum development, the improvement of postgraduate training and the introduction of retraining and continuing education programmes for existing specialists.

Funding

Funding was provided annually, following reapplication and the submission of satisfactory interim and final reports each year. The Institutional Grant (Action 1) provided support for joint training projects and covered staff costs, travel and subsistence for visits and meetings, language courses, the purchase of equipment and teaching materials, translation, printing and overheads. The Mobility Grants for staff (Action 2) covered teaching and training assignments, practical placements, retraining, updating and study periods and short visits. The total three-year grant amounted to 174 000 ECU (£125 500).

Method

There was a need to build up the infrastructure of academic equipment, including computers, software and teaching materials. A striking feature of academic departments in Hungary has been the lack of up-to-date literature and, consequently, substantial attention was given to expansion of library facilities and the acquisition of English and German textbooks and journals in child and adolescent psychiatry. Intensive language courses in English and German were set up, to facilitate access to the literature and to prepare staff for placements in Glasgow and Würzburg. Although it would have been desirable for British and German staff to have had a working knowledge of Hungarian, it was not considered practical, for the purposes of this project, to provide such language preparation.

Collaborative training activities formed the core of the project. Although the main movement was from east to west, there were two four-week teaching assignments each year to Szeged from the western centres. By the completion of the project, ten Hungarian psychiatrists, trainees or allied professionals had visited Glasgow or Würzburg, the duration of placements ranging from 4 to 33 weeks. Six British or German psychiatrists completed assignments in Szeged. In addition, the Glasgow Department's statistician held seminars and workshops in Szeged on the use of computers, statistics and research methodology.

For all placements, outline work-plans were prepared, and careful pre-planning of visits to meet various objectives was an essential requirement. All the Hungarian staff undertook one or more academic projects, participated in teaching and training, attended conferences and research meetings and received training in research techniques. In each case, individual training needs and career plans were taken into consideration and, in addition, the capacity to contribute to the activities of the host department was drawn upon as far as possible. The timing and the programme for assignments to Szeged from Glasgow and Würzburg necessitated detailed advance planning to enable optimal teaching input to be made into appropriate undergraduate and postgraduate courses, and to facilitate participation as guest lecturers in conferences of the Hungarian Association of Child Neurology and Child and Adolescent Psychiatry. Because of the language difficulties, the main input into undergraduate teaching at Szeged was in the English language curriculum, a long-established feature of the Medical University. In addition, the project coordinator met the rectors and senior academic staff at the medical universities of Budapest, Debrecen and Pécs, to discuss the necessity to develop teaching in child and adolescent psychiatry at undergraduate level.

Problems

The planning and coordination of the project was a rewarding and challenging experience, although not without numerous day-to-day administrative and organisational difficulties. The clarification and harmonising of reciprocal expectations between the three centres was a recurrent critical issue, requiring regular communication between the project leaders. This reflects the fact that both before and after successful bids for funding for such international collaborative projects, the nominated coordinator needs to make a detailed on-site evaluation of training requirements, and of the capacity of partner centres either to benefit from participation or make appropriate response to the identified needs. Such information is an essential preliminary for preparing detailed work-plans for both short- and long-term placements, in order to meet diverse individual and institutional training requirements.

Despite substantial investment in language preparation, language difficulties continued to pose a significant problem, especially since psychiatry relies so heavily on effective verbal and written communication. This was one of the factors complicating participant observation in clinical work and access to patients in the three centres, in addition to the restrictions imposed by the licensing procedures for foreign doctors on brief visits to Germany and the UK.

Initially, when the policy was to buy most equipment in the UK, the selection, supply and installation of equipment posed repeated problems. As the project progressed, however, it became preferable, both practically and economically, to purchase most equipment in Hungary. Finally, despite intensive efforts involving many hours of meetings, only limited progress has been made in establishing recognition of child and adolescent psychiatry in the priorities of the medical universities, other than at Szeged, and it remains unclear how far any lasting institutional changes have been achieved.

Benefits for Hungary

Despite transient difficulties, all participants are in no doubt that the project has made a substantial contribution to developments in Hungary. Opportunities for increased information and awareness and for the internationalisation of practice have been available for all teaching staff in child and adolescent psychiatry at Szeged. The teaching infrastructure has been improved substantially and the facilitation of innovative change has been striking. Enhanced speciality status of child and adolescent psychiatry has been associated with increased undergraduate teaching time (currently eight hours of lectures and six hours of practical experience) and curriculum development. There is growing awareness of the need to reduce the clinical commitments of academic staff to allow more time for teaching and research, despite the persistent lack of adequate manpower, and the possibility of a chair in child and adolescent psychiatry has been considered.

A major TEMPUS initiative in the final year was the preparation of the first textbook in child and adolescent psychiatry to be written in Hungarian, an approach which is believed to have greater merit than the translation of existing Western texts. This involved substantial editorial work and the active collaboration of many personnel who had had limited or no previous experience of undertaking academic writing. Such activities have enhanced the sense of corporate identity of child and adolescent psychiatrists working in different parts of Hungary, and have provided a real opportunity for updating and continuing education. Finally, as research funds begin to be made available in Hungary, it is encouraging that several applications from child and adolescent psychiatry have been successful already.

Benefits for EC departments and universities

Involvement in such projects is time-consuming, especially for the coordinator, and it is essential that intending participants give full consideration to the potential benefits and disadvantages for Western partners.

Although there are no financial advantages attached to TEMPUS projects for EC departments or universities, there have been a number of other direct and indirect benefits.

First and foremost was the beneficial effect of participating in a funded project concerned with developing teaching and training. In itself, this is a rarity, since grant income usually flows into research, leaving teaching and training to compete with demands of clinical work and allowing educational achievements to go unrewarded. At a time of increasing pressure for quality assurance in UK university teaching, this project has been timely. The expansion of international professional contacts and the broadening of academic horizons have contributed directly to staff development at all levels in both participating EC departments. A number of innovative projects have been generated, including in Glasgow a computerised induction programme for ICD–10 and a survey of child and adolescent psychiatry teaching in medical schools throughout Europe, which has attracted the support of all the international associations concerned with medical education. Unfortunately, in the UK, despite the intense competitiveness to obtain a TEMPUS grant and the academic rigour of the work entailed, the project does not count as an academic performance indicator, or as the equivalent of research income for university funding purposes.

Although, quite explicitly, research is not funded by the TEMPUS programme, the new international links have laid the foundations of long-term scientific research collaboration between the three centres, with possibilities of involvement in wider projects concerned with the mental health implications of the current rapid social, economic and political changes.

Finally, it is likely that the enhanced international profile of the EC departments will serve to attract staff and students to these locations and to the speciality, giving long-term benefits to the universities. The University of Glasgow, for example, has been particularly successful in attracting EC grants and east European studies and initiatives are thriving.

Conclusions

The next few years will be marked by increasing emphasis on the harmonisation of standards in undergraduate and postgraduate medical education in all countries of the EC, and by growing pressure from central and eastern Europe for material and professional support to restructure training and clinical services and to assure continuing collaboration. In this context, the programme described in this chapter is offered as a workable model for future international partnerships in psychiatric training.

Although most TEMPUS JEPs are larger, involving multiple universities and higher training organisations, the small scale of this project has facilitated the development of valuable close personal contacts. For this reason, numerous requests from other centres to join the project have had to be rejected. In addition to these approaches, advice has been sought from the project coordinator by a considerable number of central and eastern European psychiatrists about the establishment of contact with Western colleagues likely to be interested in collaboration and exchange. East–west communication networks in child and adolescent psychiatry have been slow to develop, and a form of contact information service, therefore, is needed urgently to provide details of individuals and clinical or academic centres with a declared interest in cooperative training or research projects.

The development of such activities calls for concerted action in the promotion of academic links and new funding programmes by national professional bodies (e.g. the Royal College of Psychiatrists), European associations (such as the European Society for Child and Adolescent Psychiatry), and international organisations (including the International Association for Child and Adolescent Psychiatry and Allied Professions (IACAPAP) and the World Health Organization). For existing specialists and trainee psychiatrists from the former Eastern Bloc countries, the overriding necessity, currently, is for opportunities to be provided in Western European centres to experience different theoretical models and advanced clinical practice, and to be able to observe and participate in comprehensive teaching and training programmes. While the scientific basis of training, clinical practice and research has much in common across international boundaries, it is essential to acknowledge and encourage adaptation to local and national cultural standards and needs. At the present time, Western centres enjoy the advantage of greater academic and material resources but, nevertheless, the emphasis in all collaborative schemes should rest on partnership and on the quest for reciprocal benefits.

References

TEMPUS (1992a) *Scheme for Cooperation and Mobility in Higher Education Between Central/Eastern Europe and the European Community. Guide for Applicants (Vademecum), Academic Year 1993/94.* Brussels: Commission of the European Communities.
—— (1992b) *Compendium 1991/92.* Brussels: Commission of the European Communities.

Part VI. Attitudes to mental illness

17 Tolerance of mental illness in Europe

PETER HALL, IAN BROCKINGTON, MARTIN EISEMANN and MICHAEL MADIANOS

The increasing worldwide discharge of formerly institutionalised mentally ill patients into the community, and the increasing focus on alternatives to the traditional large psychiatric hospital, have obvious ethical, clinical, financial, logistic and political implications. With the consequently increased contact between severely disabled mentally ill patients and the general population, their relatives, and community agencies, neglect of the limits of community tolerance could have adverse effects on the patients and even on the mental health of the wider community. There could also be backfiring, putting efforts to develop community care into jeopardy and increasing rather than decreasing the stigma of mental illness.

There has been no real mandate from the community at large for these changes in mental health practice. The community may not be capable of showing the skills and tolerance which were previously the province of the mental hospital and its staff. Tolerance has to be distinguished from indifference, and intolerance also has to be distinguished from a legitimate reaction to the all-too-common lack of adequate provision in community based programmes.

The World Health Organization (WHO), being aware of the paucity of European research on this topic (Bhugra, 1989), organised a workshop in Umea, Sweden, in March 1985 to discuss the whole question in depth, in the hope of launching collaborative research in the various countries concerned. There proved to be some felicitous overlap between studies conducted in Greece, Sweden, Italy and the UK, which will be discussed later.

Previous studies

North American studies have reached conflicting results; for example, Cumming & Cumming (1957) found that public attitudes were those of denial, isolation and insulation of mental illness, or "that the greatest obstacle to community care is the pervasive hostility to acceptance of the mentally ill in many communities" (Gorman, 1976). Others had found that the patients' actual experiences seemed more benign.

Farina & Ring (1965) concluded that the majority of patients in psychiatric hospitals are not seriously concerned with questions of stigma, and Swanson & Spitzer (1970) came to similar conclusions about patients' relatives. Freeman & Simmons (1965) reported that about a quarter of relatives had concerns about stigma, but that this related principally to difficult problems of behaviour when patients remained overtly unwell. Gove & Fain (1973) found that a minority of ex-patients were initially embarrassed or uncomfortable about having been in a psychiatric hospital, but did not perceive stigma as having long-term consequences. Angermeyer *et al* (1987) suggested that patients discharged from modern treatment settings actually perceived more stigma than those patients who had been discharged from a more traditional institution.

Ross & Ashok (1983) studied attitudes in teenagers and found that girls tended to be more socially accepting than boys. Yamamoto & Dizney (1967) carried out a study among student teachers and found that individuals were increasingly rejected if described as needing the help of a clergyman, physician, psychiatrist or mental hospital, and that social behaviour rather than severity of symptoms determined the degree of rejection.

An unpublished study was carried out in India by Roy comparing urban and village attitudes and found – surprisingly – that the village population was more tolerant of mental illness, felt that it was due to illness and would go to hospital rather than a temple. Shurka (1983) found that, in Israel, patients themselves expressed very negative feelings towards other patients, and much more positive feelings towards people perceived as normal. Daseberg *et al* (1984) carried out a survey of three low-income, high-density suburbs of Jerusalem and found that about two-thirds of their respondents thought the mentally ill could do a job well, and almost all of them supported community-based services.

Cohen & Stroenig (1962) found that psychiatrists were most socially restrictive of mentally ill patients, and that psychologists were very little better.

As well as these individual papers, there have been several excellent reviews. Firstly, Stephen Segal (1978) concluded that the public view a broader range of behaviour as mental illness than they used to, that the pattern of behaviour is the major determinant, and that there is little evidence of a direct relationship between the negative attitudes held by the public and their behaviour towards the mentally ill. In a later paper, Segal *et al* (1980) suggests that social class is vital and that conservative middle-class communities are the most negative in attitude. Conservative working-class neighbourhoods are intermediate, and non-traditional neighbourhoods are "close to the ideal accepting community".

A more recent review which deserves to be more widely known is that by Sellick & Goodyear (1985), who surveyed three large rural areas in Australia, and found that older, less educated members of the public are more positive in their opinions about mental illness.

Kirby & James (1979) carried out a comparative study of Australian, British and Czechoslovak doctors' attitudes, and found that European doctors were much less tolerant than Australian ones. There was also interesting correspondence in the *Psychiatric Bulletin* of the Royal College of Psychiatrists about *Stigma and the Psychiatric Patient* (Turner, 1986), and the fourth Collegiate Trainees Committee of the College (Bhugra & Scott, 1989) carried out a pilot study of *The Public Image of Psychiatry*, which circulated questionnaires among general practitioner surgery attenders, on the basis that public attitudes to the mentally ill were generally rejecting and anxious. They found that men were more likely to object to a hostel for the mentally ill in their street, but nearly a fifth of respondents felt that the mentally ill were non-violent, while an overwhelming majority thought that the mentally ill were "inadequate". Almost two-thirds saw mental illness like any other illness, and less than half of women and a third of men saw mental illness as a disturbance of the nervous system. Almost all of the respondents felt that mental hospitals were necessary, but only about a tenth felt that these should be away from towns or relatives, and most respondents felt they should not have guards or fences and that wards should be open.

Among the very few European studies, a useful and seemingly little-known study in Edinburgh (McClean, 1968) suggested that people were generally tolerant and well informed, and that high tolerance was related to youth, relatively good education and social class, and to a high score for neuroticism on the short scale of the Maudsley Personality Inventory.

Scott *et al* (1983) interviewed 400 residents of Tucson, Arizona, and Dabbin *et al* (1984) conducted a telephone survey of three New York boroughs, and found that most living within a street or two of psychiatric facilities were unaware of their existence. Flasberod & Kuiz (1983) carried out a mailed questionnaire in Illinois, Indiana, Michigan, Minnesota, Ohio and Wisconsin, and found that rural attitudes were more tolerant than in the city.

Nieradzyk & Cochrane (1985) found in a small but important study in Birmingham that public attitudes to mental illnesses were rejecting, more so if behaviour was disturbed and/or if the individual had been labelled as mentally ill. They concluded that negative attitudes were not related to social class.

The most recent review of the literature is by Bhugra (1989) who gives a useful bibliography of over 100 references and considers that – unlike those in the US – "European attitudes towards mental illness have risen from the Athenian thinking on the psyche". He also echoes the pessimism of several other writers about changing attitudes by health education. There are also older classic reviews, for example by Taylor *et al* (1979), Rabkin (1972), Johannsen (1969), Cohen & Stroenig (1962), Nunnally (1961) and Phillips (1964). Link (1985) and Link *et al* (1985) have also written about attitudes to mental illness as part of "labelling" theory.

Methodology

The WHO conference revealed a number of relevant European studies. Swedish (Umea) and Italian (Naples) studies looked at 1081 and 945 individuals respectively, aged between 16 and 74 years. Selection was by multistep random sampling with optimal stratification. The socio-demographic variables taken into account were: sex; age; educational level; social class; area of residence; and previous contact with the mentally ill.

In the Greek study (Madianos *et al*, 1987), 1574 men and women resident in the Greater Athens area were studied, using a two-stage systematic sampling procedure (giving a 15% sample of the total number of households), and interviewing one adult member aged 19–64 years from each household using a Kish selection grid (Kish, 1965). The instrument used was the Opinion About Mental Illness Scale (Cohen & Stroenig, 1962).

In the Worcester (UK) study, 1987 people were interviewed, selected by quota sampling (i.e. interviewing one person per household from a random sample of census enumeration districts, each containing 150–200 households). The demographic features used in the study were similar to the previous ones mentioned. The instrument used was largely derived from Cohen & Stroenig's scale, but as modified by Link (1985). Considerable further modification of the Cohen & Stroenig (1962) scale was necessary to try to eliminate possible bias and duplication, to remove statements which appeared to assume medical knowledge, to allow for 'don't know' categories, to allow some statements to be replaced by attitudinal ones, and to equalise the number of questions worded negatively as opposed to positively. This resulted in 31 statements about respondents' attitudes to mental illness.

Results

Of 27 questions asked in the Swedish and Italian studies, 51 questions in the Greek, and 31 in the British study, 11 questions can be regarded as roughly comparable.

Although the comparability of these 11 particular questions (Tables 17.1 and 17.2) is somewhat fortuitous, the full analysis of the UK study (Cronbachs Alpha to validate, and principal component factor analysis)

TABLE 17.1
Responses to questions posed on attitudes to the mentally ill in Sweden, Italy, Greece and the UK

Questions	Sweden %	Italy %	Greece %	UK %
1. Only people with a weak psyche develop mental illnesses. One of the main causes of mental illness is a lack of moral strength and willpower.	8	58	68	19
2. More taxes should be spent on severe mental illness.	57	62	94	78
3. Mentally ill people scare me. They are far more of a danger than most suppose. It is dangerous to forget for a moment that they are mentally ill, although they may seem all right.	27	65	63	8
4. A mentally ill person can do a skilled job of work.	67	20	58	65
5. I might marry a person who has been mentally ill.	33	13	37	5
6. Anyone can become mentally ill.	90	31	34	88
7. The mentally ill should be isolated in mental hospitals away from the rest of the community.	24	33	12	5
8. See Table 17.2.				
9. I would not mind living next door to someone who is mentally ill.	72	43	—	55
10. I would not mind living near a treatment centre for the mentally ill.	77	21	—	70
11. It is best for the mentally ill to be treated/live in the community.	53	48	—	72

yielded three main factors (Brockington *et al*, 1993). In that study, factor 1 was concerned with fear of the mentally ill, and in this comparative study, question 3 had the highest factorial loading on that factor (– 0.69). The second factor in Brockington *et al* (1993) had to do with personal exclusion from closeness, and in the factorial analysis, question 5 had the highest loading (+ 0.56). The third factor concerned general 'benevolence' (what previous workers have called "mental health ideology"). In that factor, question 2 of this study was the third most important (+ 0.47).

The 11 questions of this international comparison are, therefore, fairly crucial, and to set them in context, in factor 1, age (65 or more) was the next most important factor (at only + 0.13). So far as factor 2 was concerned, age was again the next most important feature (+ 0.53). In factor 3, the most important feature was education over the age of 25 (at + 0.41), with 'working with the mentally ill' second (+ 0.34).

TABLE 17.2

Question 8: "Have you been in touch with somebody who is, or has been mentally ill?"

	Naples (Italy)	Umea (Sweden)	Malvern (UK)	Bromsgrove (UK)	Athens (Greece)
n	945	1081	1000	987	1574
No	45%	21%	33.4%	26.4%	32.0%
Don't know	3%	2%	0	0.5%	0.1%
Self	N/A	N/A	6.6%	5.9%	5.7%
Family member	} 13%	} 27%	25.4%	25.9%	} 3.6%
Other relative			10.1%	13%	
Friend	N/A	N/A	28.9%	31.9%	} 30.1%
Acquaintance	50%	44%	13.3%	12.6%	

In question 1 there appears to be a clear north/south Europe divide. The opposite question 6 is consistent as it shows the opposite. It is interesting that in the question of whether more tax money should be spent on the mentally ill, this north/south divide does not appear to exist. This may, of course, reflect the existing tax structures. In question 3, as to whether the mentally ill are frightening or not, only 8% of the UK respondents said they were, with Sweden second at 27%, and Greece and Italy very similar at approximately 65%. This is reflected in the question of whether community-based psychiatric facilities are best, where the UK again gave the highest level of positive response at 72%, Sweden 53% and Italy 48%. Question 7 (that mental hospitals are the best place of treatment) produced complementary responses (UK 5%, Sweden 24%, Greece 12%, Italy 33%). It would appear that although in some ways the Swedish respondents seem the most tolerant, the UK respondents express very little fear of the mentally ill, a feeling that almost anyone could become mentally ill, a rejection of closed mental hospitals, and a mandate for community-based facilities.

On the issue of possible marriage to a person who has been mentally ill, Sweden has the surprisingly high score of 33%, Italy very much less at 13%, Greece (where the question was admittedly somewhat different) 37% and the UK (where the question was the same as the Greek one) 5%. It is perhaps relevant that in another part of the study (Hall *et al*, 1993) where vignettes of clearly very disturbed people were shown to respondents, 3–5% of the UK respondents stated that they might be prepared to marry the subject (slightly more among males).

It is also interesting to look at question 4 which relates to the work capacity of the mentally ill. More than 60% of the respondents from Greece, Sweden and the UK agreed that the mentally ill were able to work satisfactorily in many cases, despite their mental illness. The Italian respondents scored only 20%, for reasons that are far from clear.

In the question of the acceptability of the mentally ill as neighbours, there were similar results for all three countries (43–72%). This contrasted with question 10 (the desirability of locating mental health treatment facilities in the community), where Sweden and the UK gave similar positive responses, but Italy was quite different at 21%. Perhaps Italian patients are less inhibited, but it is a particular pity that this question was not included in the Greek study.

In the UK detailed statistical analysis, those who knew someone who had been mentally ill compared with those who knew no-one showed increased tolerance on all statements (Table 17.2) to a high degree of statistical significance, and also showed a pronounced gradient depending on the closeness of the known person. There was also a tendency for tolerance to increase depending on the closeness of the friendship, but to decrease if the mentally ill person was a member of the respondent's actual family. Those who had personally experienced mental illness were less tolerant than those who knew someone with mental illness (and, indeed, even those with no personal experience).

In the full UK analysis, the most generally tolerant were those of higher education and the younger individuals (older people were markedly less tolerant). The other most important factor regarding tolerance was social class, where higher social classes were almost invariably more tolerant than lower social classes, as were those working with the mentally ill. (Interestingly, though, those working with the mentally ill in the UK showed less tolerance in the question suggesting that more tax money should be spent on their clients.)

Clearly one should not read too much into these studies, as it is difficult to compare Naples or Athens with a small English town or with Sweden. Nevertheless, the questions are topical, seem important, and it is interesting to compare the countries concerned and to make what one will of the data, such as they are.

References and further reading

ANGERMEYER, M. C., LINK, B. & MAJCHER-ANGERMEYER, A. (1987) Stigma perceived by patients attending modern treatment settings. *Journal of Nervous and Mental Disease*, **175**, 4–11.

AVIRAM, U. & SEGAL, S. P. (1973) Exclusion of the mentally ill. *Archives of General Psychiatry*, **29**, 126–131.

BHUGRA, D. (1989) Attitudes towards mental illness – a review. *Acta Psychiatrica Scandinavica*, **80**, 1–12.

—— & SCOTT, J. (1989) The public image of psychiatry (pilot study). *Bulletin of the Royal College of Psychiatrists*, January, 330–331.

BROCKINGTON, I. A., HALL, P., LEVINGS, J. J., *et al* (1993) Tolerance of the mentally ill in two West Midland communities. *British Journal of Psychiatry*, **162**, 93–99.

CARPENTER, J. O. & BOURESTOM, N. C. (1976) Performance of psychiatric hospital discharges in strict and tolerant environments. *Community Mental Health Journal*, **12**, 45–51.

COHEN, J. & STROENIG, E. L. (1962) Opinions about mental illness in the personnel of two large mental hospitals. *Journal of Abnormal and Social Psychology*, **64**, 349–360.

CROCETTI, G., SPIRO, H. R. & SIASSI, I. (1971) Are the ranks closed? Attitude and social distance and mental illness. *American Journal of Psychiatry*, **127**, 1121–1127.

CUMMING, E. & CUMMING, J. (1957) *An Experiment in Mental Health: Closed Ranks*. Cambridge, MA: Harvard University Press.

DABBIN, J., MUHLIN, G. & COHEN, P. (1984) What the neighbours think: community attitudes towards local psychiatric facilities. *Community Health Journal*, **20**, 305–311.

DASEBERG, H., SHEFLER, G., PAYNTON, N., *et al* (1984) Local attitudes as a basis for the planning of a community mental health service in Jerusalem. *Israel Journal of Psychiatry and Related Science*, **4**, 247–265.

DEPARTMENT OF HEALTH AND SOCIAL SECURITY (1970) *A Feasibility Study for a Model Reorganisation of Mental Illness Services*. London: HMSO.

FARINA, A. & RING, K. (1965) The influence of perceived mental illness on interpersonal relations. *Journal of Abnormal Psychology*, **70**, 47–51.

FLASBEROD, J. & KUIZ, F. (1983) Rural attitudes and knowledge of mental illness and treatment resources. *Hospital and Community Psychiatry*, **8**, 229–233.

FREEMAN, H. E. & SIMMONS, O. G. (1965) Feelings of stigma among relatives of former mental patients. *Social Problems*, **8**, 312–321.

GORMAN, M. (1976) Community absorption of the mentally ill: the new challenge. *Community Mental Health Journal*, **12**, 119–127.

GOVE, W. & FAIN, T. (1973) The stigma of mental hospitalisation. *Archives of General Psychiatry*, **22**, 494–500.

HALL, P. & GILLARD, R. (1982) The Worcester Development Project. *International Journal of Social Psychiatry*, **28**, 163–172.

———, BROCKINGTON, I. F., MURPHY, C. J., *et al* (1990) *Tolerance of the Mentally Ill in Two West Midland Communities*. Unpublished report to the Health Promotion Research Trust.

———, ———, LEVINGS, J., *et al* (1993) A comparison of responses to the mentally ill in two communities. *British Journal of Psychiatry*, **162**, 99–108.

HARNOIS, G., COVIN, E., UCHOA, E., *et al* (1989) *Attitudes in the Field of Mental Health – Theoretical & Methodological Guidelines*. Unpublished report to the World Health Organization by the WHO Collaborating Centre (Montreal).

HASSALL, C. (1982) *Comparison of United Kingdom Case Registers*. Unpublished report, University of Birmingham.

JOHANNSEN, W. J. (1969) Attitudes towards mental patients. A review of empirical research. *Mental Health Hygiene*, **53**, 218–228.

KIRBY, R. J. & JAMES, R. A. (1979) Attitudes of medical practitioners to mental illness. *Australian and New Zealand Journal of Psychiatry*, **13**, 165–168.

KISH, L. (1965) *Survey Sampling*. New York: John Wiley.

LINK, B. (1985) The labelling perspective and its critics. A reformulation in the area of mental disorder. Paper presented to the Eastern Sociological Association Meeting, Philadelphia.

———, CULLEN, F., STROENIG, E., *et al* (1985) A modified labelling approach to mental disorders. Unpublished report, Columbia University, USA.

McCLEAN, U. (1968) The 1966 Edinburgh survey of community attitudes to mental illness. *Health Bulletin*, **25**, 1–5.

MADIANOS, M. G., MADIANOU, D., VLACHONIKOLIS, J., *et al* (1987) Attitudes towards mental illness in the Athens area. *Acta Psychiatrica Scandinavica*, **75**, 158–165.

NIERADZYK, K. & COCHRANE, R. (1985) Public attitudes towards mental illness, the effect of behaviour and psychiatric labels. *International Journal of Social Psychiatry*, **31**, 23–33.

NUNNALLY, J. (1961) *Popular Conceptions of Mental Health, Their Development and Change*. New York: Holt, Rinehart & Winston.

PHILLIPS, D. L. (1964) Rejection of the mentally ill: the influence of behaviour and sex. *American Sociological Review*, **5**, 679–687.

RABKIN, J. G. (1972) Opinions about mental illness. *Psychological Bulletin*, **77**, 153–171.

ROSS, M. G. N. & ASHOK, K. M. (1983) Adolescents' attitudes towards mental illness. *Social Psychiatry*, **18**, 45–60.

SCOTT, R., BALCH, P. & FLYNN, T. (1983) A comparison of community attitudes towards CMCC services with those of a mental hospital. *American Journal of Community Psychology*, **2**, 741–745.

SEGAL, S. (1978) Attitudes towards the mentally ill – a review. *Social Work*, May, 211–217.

———, BAUMOHL, J. & MAYLES, E. (1980) Neighourhood types and community reaction to the mentally ill. *Journal of Health and Social Behaviour*, **21**, 345–359.

SELLICK, K. & GOODYEAR, J. (1985) Community attitudes towards mental illness – the influence of contact and demographic variables. *Australian and New Zealand Journal of Psychiatry*, **19**, 293–298.

SHURKA, E. (1983) The evaluation of ex-mental patients by other ex-mental patients. *International Journal of Social Psychiatry*, **29**, 286–291.

SWANSON, R. & SPITZER, S. (1970) Stigma and the psychiatric patient's career. *Journal of Health and Social Behaviour*, **11**, 44–51.

TAYLOR, S. M., DEAR, M. J. & HALL, G. B. (1979) Attitudes towards the mentally ill and reactions to mental health facilities. *Social Science and Medicine*, **13**, 281–290.

TURNER, T. H. (1986) Stigma and the psychiatric patient. *Bulletin of the Royal College of Psychiatry*, **10**, 8 & 359.

YAMAMOTO, K. & DIZNEY, H. (1967) Rejection of the mentally ill. *Journal of Counselling Psychology*, **14**, 264–268.

18 Schisms in European psychiatry

**JIM VAN OS, PALOMA GALDOS,
GLYN LEWIS, MARK BOURGEOIS
and ANTHONY MANN**

Economic and political union are high on the agenda in the European Union (EU), and medical doctors can work in any of the member states, the prospect of which enthuses some (Smith, 1991), but generates apprehension in others (Appleby, 1988). It is becoming increasingly clear that there are widespread differences in medical practice in Europe, not only in psychiatry, but also in areas ranging from the diagnosis of low blood pressure (Wessely *et al*, 1990) to the treatment of testicular cancer (Stoter, 1987). If the implementation of European union is to be applied to the field of medicine as well, then medical practitioners in the member states will have to create consensus in areas of disagreement.

Psychiatrists in the UK have been keen to examine international differences in psychiatric practice. For instance, one of the high points of epidemiological psychiatry was the comparison of diagnostic habits between US and UK psychiatrists (Cooper *et al*, 1972). In the 1960s, large and persistent differences existed between the diagnostic statistics generated by American and British psychiatric hospitals. Some years later, Cooper *et al* (1972) concluded that these differences were mostly due to the contrasting diagnostic criteria used by American and British psychiatrists, despite a common language and extensive cultural and professional ties. These influential findings gave a major impetus to the standardisation of psychiatric diagnoses, culminating in the development of comprehensive diagnostic rules such as the Research Diagnostic Criteria (Spitzer *et al*, 1978).

Within Europe, however, psychiatric traditions seem to be more resistant to such consensus formation, and it would appear that the traditional divide between Anglo-Saxon empiricism and continental rationalism – trying to reach the truth through experiment or through ideas – has affected psychiatric practice. This is perhaps epitomised by the psychiatric traditions of the UK and France. We will review, in this chapter, the main disparities in psychiatric practice in these two countries, and analyse them in light of the European union now taking place.

Diagnosis and administrative incidence

Since the above-mentioned US/UK study demonstrated that differences in diagnostic practice result in differences in the incidence of psychiatric disorders as recorded by national hospital admission statistics, contrasting diagnostic habits have become a regular topic in psychiatric 'transcultural' research.

In the UK, the Kraepelinian dichotomy has survived until today, with the category of 'other psychoses' to accommodate those psychotic disorders not considered clearly affective or schizophrenic. The ICD–9 category 'paranoid states' (ICD 297) is traditionally considered part of the schizophrenic spectrum in the UK (Kendell, 1987), and is combined with schizophrenic disorders in national mental health statistics. In France, diagnostic practice appears more refined, not unlike DSM–III–R (Pull *et al*, 1987; Kellam, 1989). Apart from schizophrenia and manic–depressive psychoses, separate categories exist to accommodate acute, good-outcome, non-affective psychotic states (*psychoses délirantes aiguës-bouffée délirante*), and the delusional disorders (*délires chroniques*). The Heboïdophrenic (pseudopsychopathic) schizophrenia subtype is encountered in psychiatric textbooks in France (Lemperière & Féline, 1983), but it is not recognised in the UK.

It is therefore not surprising that comparative investigations found that there was considerable variation in diagnostic conventions among European psychiatrists. Kendall *et al* (1974), using video-taped interviews, found that French and English psychiatrists differed markedly in their concept of psychiatric disorder, especially affective illness. A casenote study by Johnson-Sabine *et al* (1983) examined the French diagnostic concept of *bouffée délirante*, and found that it did not correspond to any orthodox British diagnostic category when cases were rediagnosed by UK psychiatrists. However, all these studies focused on small and unrepresentative samples of European psychiatrists, and did not try to link results to epidemiological data.

In a recent study (Van Os *et al*, 1993) a questionnaire was sent to a random sample of 240 psychiatrists in the two countries (response rate: 74%), asking them about their opinions regarding the aetiology, diagnosis and management of schizophrenia. The questionnaire consisted of 38 statements with a seven-point Likert scale (midpoint 4), anchored at both ends between agreement and disagreement. Highly significant differences were found for 33 of the 38 statements; in 11 instances, the mean score indicated that psychiatrists in the two countries actually disagreed with each other.

French psychiatrists reserved the label schizophrenia for disorders with onset before age 45, a chronic course and poor outcome (*état déficitaire*), although French psychiatrists, but not their British counterparts, on average also agreed that mixed affective and schizophrenic states – generally associated with a more benign course of illness – should be included in the concept. The French sample regarded dissociation and discordance as the key symptoms, and had a 'pseudopsychopathic' subtype of schizophrenia, which is not recognised by the British. In the UK, good outcome and late-onset cases tended to be included, as well as chronic delusional or hallucinatory states without personality deterioration. Schneider's first rank symptoms were considered core features. These differences are impressive, especially with respect to core symptomatology. Dissociation and discordance in general refer to abnormalities of the associative processes, abnormalities of affect, and ambivalence (Lanteri-Laura, 1981). Symptoms such as these are not really clear cut, and the sort of diagnostic deliberation that leads to their detection in France is likely to differ considerably from that performed by UK psychiatrists. For instance, in our questionnaire study, the French sample agreed that Rorschach's projection test was a useful tool in establishing the diagnosis of schizophrenia; the British, however, strongly disagreed.

It seems likely that some of these differences will be reflected in the administrative incidence (first admissions) of schizophrenia in the two countries. A comparison of first admission rates to psychiatric hospitals and units in France and England over the period 1973–1982 (Van Os *et al*, 1993) demonstrated that the rates in France showed a marked decline after the age of 45, whereas in England they continued to rise, especially in women. This decline of first admission rates in France after the age of 45 is consistent with the replies given in the questionnaire survey. Before the age of 45, first admission rates in France were much higher for both men and women. Evidence from the questionnaire survey suggested, on the one hand, that French diagnostic criteria were narrower, as schizophrenia was viewed as a chronic syndrome resulting in deterioration, with exclusion of acute onset and good outcome cases. However, the French regarded the less clearly defined Bleulerian signs (Bleuler, 1911; Pichot, 1982) as the key symptoms of the disorder, reminiscent of the situation in the US before the advent of standardised criteria. Also, the French had a subtype of schizophrenia, not recognised by the British. It appeared, therefore, that the French concept of schizophrenia encompassed a variety of chronic states, which would have been excluded in the UK for lack of specific symptomatology. Although it is possible that the observed differences reflected differences in real incidence (Der *et al*, 1990), it is probable that more than one mechanism was involved, and diagnostic bias was a likely one (for a discussion, see Van Os *et al*, 1993). Unless operationalised criteria are applied retrospectively to all cases, comparison of first admission rates between the two countries for epidemiological research is impossible at present.

Theories of aetiology

As there is a large degree of *non-savoir* as to what constitutes the causes of psychiatric disorders, it is likely that the local cultural climate will influence the way in which psychiatric professionals attempt to fill the gaps. In the UK, psychiatry has enjoyed a close relationship with traditional medicine, and strict application of the scientific method is the rule. On the continent, and especially in France, psychoanalysis has been much more influential (*Le Monde*, 1982), and this may have had an effect on theories of aetiology.

The influence of Jacques Lacan may serve as an example. This psychoanalyst has been considered the mainspring of the "invasion of French intellectual life by psychoanalysis" (Turkle, 1978), and has had a profound influence on the conceptualisation and psychoanalytic treatment of psychosis in French psychiatry. Lacan published his first book in 1966, and his influence in France greatly increased throughout the 1970s and early 1980s. The Lacanian outlook included the linguistic structure of the unconscious and linked with mathematics, resulting in a highly complicated and speculative study of the interpretation of verbal forms and phonemic structure, and numerical formulations of transition processes, which serve to generate mathematical models (Miller, 1987). Lacan, for all his popularity in France and elsewhere, appears to have been largely ignored in the UK. Our questionnaire survey provided support for this. For instance, French psychiatrists on average agreed strongly with the statement that the language of schizophrenic patients reflects unconscious processes, and considered that recognition of these was an important therapeutic aid. British psychiatrists on average did not accept this.

To get a better impression of the currently prevailing theories in the UK and France, we included in our questionnaire survey several questions regarding the aetiology of schizophrenia. This revealed marked divergence in almost all statements. French psychiatrists favoured psychoanalytically-orientated aetiological statements, such as absence of the paternal image and maternal ambivalence during childhood, while their British counterparts scored high on items postulating neurodevelopmental and genetic causation. The fact that schizophrenia tends to affect several members in the same extended family was considered a genetic effect by the British, but the French on average preferred an environmental, or 'pseudogenetic' interpretation. There were also striking differences regarding the role of family dynamics and parental factors in the causation of schizophrenia, French psychiatrists giving much more importance to these than their British colleagues.

Treatment issues

In the UK, the acquisition of psychotherapeutic skills during psychiatric training has low priority compared with other EU countries (Van Beinum, 1993). This may affect treatment strategies for psychiatric disorders, and also create contrasting patient expectations.

It appears that disparities in the management of disorders are not confined to psychotherapy alone. For instance, Deniker's (1983) classification of antipsychotics into incisive, alerting and sedating subtypes in France does not appear to be recognised in the UK, which presumably indicates that there may be differences in the clinical use of these compounds in the two countries.

Our questionnaire survey supported these impressions. The British sample almost invariably indicated disagreement with psychoanalytical statements, in favour of biological and behavioural theory. For instance, British psychiatrists on average rejected psychoanalytical psychotherapy, and the French rejected behavioural psychotherapy in the treatment of schizophrenia. They also gave different views regarding the use and properties of antipsychotic medication. French psychiatrists had more distinctive indications for different antipsychotics, especially in the treatment of aggressive behaviour and negative symptoms. Probably as a consequence, they showed a preference for treating patients with more than one kind of antipsychotic compound, which was disapproved of by the British. Interestingly, in France, psychiatrists saw a more important role for the hospital than in Britain, but then the British group appeared much more frustrated with the perceived inadequacy of community services. French psychiatrists, in making a decision to admit a patient involuntarily, appeared to focus more on individual suffering than their British counterparts.

Conclusions

It could be argued that French and English psychiatry lie at opposite ends of the European continuum, and that differences between other European countries would be less conspicuous. Our argument, however, is that psychiatric theory and practice, and – probably to a lesser extent – other disciplines in medicine, are subject to prevailing and culturally determined beliefs. We think this is important, as European doctors can now practise in any of the member states, and, as things stand now, little has been done to clear the confusion they are likely to meet when crossing the conceptual frontiers.

The divergent views on either side of the channel are in stark contrast to the attention that has been paid to transatlantic differences in psychiatric practice, and perhaps epitomise the popular reluctance regarding European union. However, in a dialectical Europe, different psychiatric traditions should be able to learn from each other, while talking in a common language. In order to achieve this, more collaborative 'transcultural' research is needed, so that psychiatrists, and – perhaps more importantly – their patients, can be enlightened, rather than perplexed, by European union.

References

APPLEBY, J. (1988) Why 1992 may be disastrous for health. *British Medical Journal*, **296**, 1620.

BLEULER, E. (1911) *Dementia Praecox or the Group of Schizophrenias* (transl. J. Zinkin, 1950). New York: International Universities Press.

COOPER, J., KENDALL, R., GURLAND, E., *et al* (1972) *Psychiatric Diagnosis in New York and London*. Maudsley Monograph No. 20. Oxford: Oxford University Press.

DENIKER, P. (1983) Discovery of the clinical use of neuroleptics. In *Discoveries in Pharmacology* (eds M. Parnham & J. Bruinvels), pp. 163–180. Amsterdam: Elsevier.

DER, G., GUPTA, S. & MURRAY, R. (1990) Is schizophrenia disappearing? *Lancet*, **335**, 513–516.

JOHNSON-SABINE, E., MANN, A., JACOBY, R., *et al* (1983) Bouffée délirante: an examination of its current status. *Psychological Medicine*, **13**, 771–778.

KELLAM, A. (1989) French empirical criteria for the diagnosis of non-affective non-organic psychoses. Comparison between the criteria suggested by Professors Pull and Pichot and those of DSM–III–R. *British Journal of Psychiatry*, **155**, 153–159.

KENDELL, R. (1987) Other functional psychoses. In *Companion to Psychiatric Studies* (eds R. Kendell & A. Zealey), pp. 362–374. Edinburgh: Churchill Livingstone.

——, PICHOT, P. & VON CRANACH, M. (1974) Diagnostic criteria of English, French, and German psychiatrists. *Psychological Medicine*, **4**, 187–195.

LANTERI-LAURA, G. (1981) Les principales théories dans la psychiatrie contemporaine. *Encycopédie Médico-Chirurgicale*, Paris, Psychiatrie, 37006 A[10.]

LE MONDE (1982) La France sur le divan. 7th March, 12.

LEMPERIÈRE, T. & FÉLINE, A. (1983) *Psychiatrie de l'Adulte*. Paris: Masson.

MILLER, G. (ed.) (1987) *Lacan*. Paris: Bordas.

PICHOT, P. (1982) The diagnosis and classification of mental disorders in French speaking countries: background, current view and comparison with other nomenclature. *Psychological Medicine*, **12**, 475–492.

PULL, M., PULL, C. & PICHOT, P. (1987) Des critères empiriques Français pour les psychoses: II. Consensus des psychiatres Français et définitions provisoires. *L'Encéphale*, **13**, 53–57.

SMITH, T. (1991) Closer links with Europe may improve standards of health care in Britain. *British Medical Journal*, **303**, 1284.

SPITZER, R., ENDICOTT, J. & ROBINS, E. (1978) Research Diagnostic Criteria: rationale and reliability. *Archives of General Psychiatry*, **35**, 773–782.

STOTER, G. (1987) Treatment strategies of testicular cancer in Europe. *International Journal of Andrology*, **10**, 407–415.

TURKLE, S. (1978) *Psychoanalytic Politics: Freud's French Revolution*. New York: Basic Books.

VAN BEINUM, M. (1993) European Trainees Conference. *Psychiatric Bulletin*, **17**, 96–97.

VAN OS, J., GALDOS, P., LEWIS, G., *et al* (1993) Schizophrenia sans frontières. *British Medical Journal*, **307**, 489–492.

WESSELY, S., NICKSON, J. & COX, B. (1990) Symptoms of low blood pressure. *British Medical Journal*, **301**, 362–365.

19 Eliciting lay beliefs about psychiatric symptoms across cultures

TOM SENSKY and GERD BAUMANN

The process by which a person comes to receive psychiatric help is complex (Goldberg & Huxley, 1980). This process most commonly starts with a decision to seek help. Help-seeking is itself influenced by a wide variety of factors (Rogler & Cortes, 1993), including the beliefs about a person's complaints or problems held by that individual and/or others. Of particular importance are the causes attributed to a given problem. Ultimately, specific causal attributions, whether regarding mental or physical symptoms, tend to be unique and may be highly idiosyncratic (Sensky, 1990). However, such beliefs and allied cognitive factors are heavily influenced by the individual's social and cultural background (Zola, 1966; Angel & Thoits, 1987; Kirmayer, 1989).

Popular lay beliefs and practices are important, because people often get advice from members of their family or other non-professionals before seeking expert help (Freidson, 1970; Furnham, 1992). Help-seeking is further complicated by the availability in some cultures of more than one tradition for managing disease or distress. For example, an epidemiological survey of an Indian village found that among those with a psychiatric disorder or epilepsy, 48% had consulted *both* a doctor *and* a traditional healer (Kapur, 1979). Unlike the experts, lay people are not necessarily concerned about models of illness or aetiology, and may be little influenced by the sometimes conflicting models used by the different experts whom they consult (Kapur, 1979).

Investigating any aspect of a culture different from one's own carries with it the problems inherent in ethnocentricity (Rack, 1982) – the interpretation of one culture using the norms of another (that of the researcher). Medicine, including psychiatry, is the product of its culture, and is therefore essentially ethnocentric (Littlewood & Lipsedge, 1986). Psychiatric nosologies are also ethnocentric, at least to some degree. Indiscriminate application of psychiatric diagnoses or even symptoms across cultures has been rightly criticised (Kleinman, 1977; Fernando, 1988;

Kirmayer, 1991). Even the term *psychiatric illness* has been renamed *human behavioural breakdown* (Fabrega, 1992).

Another problem is the definition of the group under investigation, more particularly of its cultural boundaries (Fernando, 1988). There are many definitions of culture (Leff, 1981) and of cultural boundaries (Littlewood, 1986). These definitions will always be arbitary to some degree. This is a problem for *all* medical research, not only that involving peoples of different ethnic origin. For example, within a given society, men and women may be considered culturally distinct, as may people of different social classes (Helman, 1990). However, there can be a problem in deciding whether, for example, a Hindu who has emigrated to Britain having spent his childhood in East Africa belongs to the same culture as a Hindu of the same age who migrated from India. If the latter had lived in a remote village rather than in an urban community, would this make a difference? On the other hand, Helman (1990) cautions against over-emphasising the contribution of culture to a person's symptoms or behaviour at the expense of physical or mental illness.

The ethnographic approach

Ethnography offers at least a partial solution to such difficulties. Ethnography involves describing a culture from the 'insider's' viewpoint, from the perspective of the individual being studied rather than that of the researcher. Important elements of ethnography include participant observation (Spradley, 1980) and the ethnographic interview (Spradley, 1979). The latter emphasises techniques which help the interviewer to develop an understanding of the informant's culture, and stresses the need to acquire skills in (among other things) translation competence, or the ability to translate the meanings of one culture into a form that is appropriate to another culture (Spradley, 1979).

An example – beliefs about mental problems among Asians in London

This project was carried out in west London, at a hospital whose catchment area includes a significant proportion of people of Indian or Pakistani descent. Many in the older generation migrated to Britain either directly from the Indian sub-continent or from East Africa. The study arose from the desire of psychiatrists and other health care professionals to develop a mental health service which was sensitive to the needs of the local population. Its aim was to improve the understanding by professionals of cognitive factors which could determine help-seeking.

The project developed in several stages. First, exploratory interviews were carried out with patients or ex-patients of the psychiatric unit and their families. Family members were interviewed either alone or together. The main themes explored in the interviews included common problems or complaints, perceived causes of these problems, and the sources of help (including medical and other 'experts') which had been pursued to deal with these. Descriptive data collected from these initial interviews were used to develop a more detailed, structured interview of the non-schedule type (Richardson *et al*, 1965). This was used with a further sample of patients, ex-patients and families. Care was taken to interview people of differing backgrounds – male and female, Muslim and Sikh, as well as Hindu, 'East African' and 'Asian', including people brought up in rural communities as well as those with an urban background. Selected vignettes from these interviews were transcribed and shown to a panel of 'experts' from different disciplines and with varying backgrounds (cultural spokespeople, religious leaders, etc.). The experts were asked in particular to what extent, in their opinion, the beliefs and behaviour described were typical of the cultural group to which the person being interviewed belonged.

From the descriptive information collected in this way, themes emerged about behavioural or emotional problems commonly associated with psychiatric referral or in-patient admission, about common causal attributions, and about methods of dealing with problems, either with or without expert help. These data were used in the next stage of the study, which departed from the strictly ethnographic path, to devise a questionnaire on ten of the most common problems (Fig. 19.1). Some of these problems could be recognised as equivalent to psychiatric symptoms (such as 'hears voices or strange singing' and 'has a drink problem'), while others were more general (e.g. 'lost affection for his/her spouse' and 'body feels heavy'). These problems or complaints did not, therefore, necessarily represent discrete psychiatric phenomena. As psychiatric symptoms might be ethnocentric, interpretation of information based on these might be more difficult.

The questionnaires were then administered to lay people of Asian origin in west London, the sample being gathered from non-medical settings such as large shops. Respondents, therefore, did not necessarily have previous experience of the problems asked about, or contact with mental health services. Respondents were asked, on the basis of what they would say to someone of their own sex, age and background who sought their advice about each particular problem, to indicate their own preferences from lists of attributed causes, methods of managing the problems, and experts to consult.

Data analysis

Specific techniques are available for analysing ethnographic data about attitudes or decision-making, such as decision tree modelling (Gladwin, 1989).

This is an iterative process which elicits from those making decisions (the interviewees or respondents) the criteria they use to make decisions, and these criteria are then mapped into a set of 'if–then' rules in the form of a decision tree. This is then tested on another group of respondents, and modified or elaborated as necessary. This process is said to be more akin to human decision-making, considering one dimension or category at a time, rather than methods such as probit analysis or logit analysis which operate by assigning weights to several variables (Gladwin, 1989).

Frequency data derived from studies such as the example above might be analysed using simple cross-tabulations. For example, Hindus and Muslims can be compared with respect to their causal attributions or their recommendations regarding which experts to consult. Similar comparisons can be made between any other groups where differences might be suspected, such as men versus women, rural versus urban backgrounds, and so on.

In the study described, there were 190 respondents, who answered questions on a total of 1012 problems, (each respondent was asked to respond to as many of the ten given problems as he/she wished to). Overall, across all ten problems, the most common cause attributed to the problem was 'bad treatment by the family', endorsed by 46% of the respondents, followed by 'marriage problems' (43%) and 'inside the mind' (42%). Given that the respondents (or their families, in the case of some younger respondents) had migrated to Britain, it was interesting that 25% of the respondents endorsed 'living away from home' as a cause of problems. Although using one's will-power was the most frequently endorsed advice (in 38% of the responses), other advice included seeing a specialist (36%), praying more (23%), changing diet (15%), and travelling (12%).

In this respect, significant differences emerged between those respondents who had lived in East Africa ('Africans') and those who had migrated directly from the Indian sub-continent ('Asians'). At least some of these differences persisted even when religious background or mother-tongue were controlled for. Asians were more likely than Africans to recommend prayer (40% v. 25%) or travel (21% v. 10%). Africans were more likely than Asians to suggest seeking specialist advice (37% v. 27%). This appeared to be because of the particular reluctance of older Asians to recommend seeing a specialist – only 10% recommended this, compared with 36% for the sample as a whole. Older Asians were instead more likely than others to recommend seeing a 'traditional' specialist – an Asian medical expert, or a religious expert. However, overall, a general practitioner was the specialist most frequently recommended (in 37% of responses), regardless of the problem or the cause attributed to it. In the light of Kapur's findings (mentioned above), it was of interest to examine whether respondents discriminated between traditional specialists and psychiatrists in their recommendations. These were mutually exclusive for men, in that if male respondents recommended seeing a psychiatrist, they were not likely to also recommend seeing a traditional specialist. However, this did not apply to the responses from women.

Limitations of standard data analysis

Surprisingly, few differences were found between the different problems, between Hindu and Muslim respondents, or between respondents whose parental mother-tongue was Punjabi and those for whom it was Gujarati (the two most common parental mother-tongues in the sample). However, these findings may be due to Type 2 statistical errors because, once the sample had been divided, for example, by causal attribution as well as mother-tongue, the comparisons involved smaller numbers of responses. Making particular comparisons using cross-tabulations also carries other potential problems. Selecting which comparisons to make involves hypothesis-testing. The particular hypotheses chosen might again be ethnocentric, and the results difficult to interpret. In some circumstances, however, the potential problems due to ethnocentricity might be overestimated. For example, even if the distinction between 'Africans' and 'Asians' was made by researchers or clinicians, rather than by those in the sample, it could be argued that the differences between these two groups might be clinically useful as they stand; health care workers might use these data to target education and intervention strategies for groups which can be relatively easily defined.

However, these results provide only vague answers about the reasons behind differences in beliefs and attitudes. Can the observed differences between 'Africans' and 'Asians' be accounted for by selective migration (many Africans having been forced to emigrate for political reasons), by acculturation (the prevailing culture in East Africa having been less 'traditional' than in much of India), by background (Asians who migrated to Africa were unrepresentative of Asians as a whole) or some combination of these? Even more tantalising is the possibility that the data contain relevant information which is 'hidden' because the appropriate hypotheses have not been considered, or again because of multiple variables and small cell sizes. These factors create problems not only with cross-tabulation but also with techniques such as log-linear modelling (Greenacre, 1992).

One possible solution to this problem of appropriate and effective data analysis is to use some form of non-linear multivariate analysis (Gifi, 1990), such as correspondence analysis (Greenacre, 1992). Multivariate analysis can provide a compact description of a data matrix, by aggregating data to demonstrate patterns between different variables in a simple and comprehensive way. Relationships between variables can be displayed in graphical form, as illustrated in Fig. 19.1, which shows all the problems and some of the attributed causes from the questionnaire. Variables can be

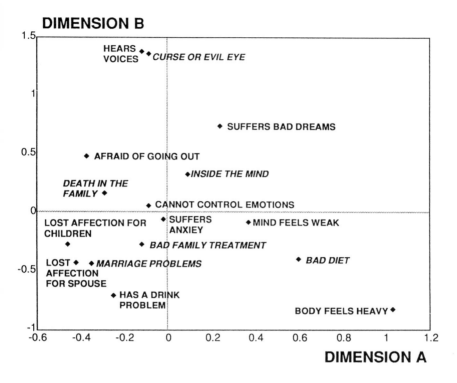

Fig. 19.1. An example of a preliminary correspondence analysis of problems (normal print) and causal attributions (italics), using homogeneity analysis for SPSS (1990).

grouped into quadrants, and by their proximity to one another on the plot. The preliminary analysis[1] in Fig. 19.1, suggests that, for example, respondents perceived 'hears voices' and 'body feels heavy' as quite different. Although relatively few respondents attributed problems to the effects of a curse, this cause mapped close to 'hears voices' in the present analysis, while 'bad diet' appeared near 'body feels heavy'.

Correspondence analysis is particularly useful in its ability to handle large data matrices, with sparse data and low sample sizes (Greenacre, 1992). Unlike commonly used inferential statistical techniques, correspondence analysis does not aim to test an *a priori* hypothesis; it is essentially *exploratory* rather than *confirmatory*. This property makes the technique particularly suitable for ethnographic data, in that the risks of ethnocentricity can be reduced.

---

1. Figure 19.1 is only illustrative and not intended as a definitive result. Analysis of the data from the study is still in progress.

Scope for further research

Ethnography may appear far removed from the experience of most psychiatrists. However, given that medicine has its own culture, most encounters with patients, if they are to be satisfactory, require doctors to have skills in translation competence and other techniques stressed by ethnographers. However, these similarities are superficial, since the objectives of medical and ethnographic interviews are different. There are also close parallels between the techniques used in ethnographic interviewing and those in cognitive therapy (Beck *et al*, 1979). Each aims to understand the interviewee's model of his or her world. Both share the fundamental principle that, with regard to this model, the interviewee is the expert. The focus of the cognitive therapist's efforts is the understanding of the individual. The ethnographer aims to understand a culture, but gathers data in the same way as the cognitive therapist, from individuals or groups. Like cognitive therapy, ethnographic interviewing uses a process of guided discovery, or Socratic questioning. The terms may be different, but their meanings are often similar. Vignettes of ethnographic interviews (Spradley, 1979) even show a clear resemblance to interviews which might be conducted by a cognitive therapist. Perhaps this is not as surprising at it may initially seem. One of the strengths of the cognitive model has been the growing relationship between cognitive therapy, which initially developed empirically, and the experimental results of cognitive psychology. Cognitive psychology has similarly influenced ethnography, whose developing methods can be seen as the results of the 'cognitive revolution' (Gladwin, 1989).

The method described of eliciting the beliefs across cultures meets at least some of the criticisms often aimed at research in transcultural psychiatry. In particular, potential problems due to ethnocentricity have been minimised by using techniques derived from ethnography, and from relatively recent developments in data analysis. Only one application of the method has been described, but similar techniques could be used successfully to examine beliefs in other cultures.

References

ANGEL, R. & THOITS, P. (1987) The impact of culture on the cognitive structure of illness. *Culture, Medicine and Psychiatry*, **11**, 465–494.

BECK, A. T., RUSH, A. J., SHAW, B. F., *et al* (1979) *Cognitive Therapy of Depression*. New York: Guilford.

FABREGA, H., Jr. (1992) The role of culture in a theory of psychiatric illness. *Social Science and Medicine*, **35**, 91–103.

FERNANDO, S. (1988) *Race, Culture and Psychiatry*. London: Croom Helm.

FREIDSON, E. (1970) *Profession of Medicine: A Study of the Sociology of Applied Knowledge*. New York: Russell Sage Foundation.

FURNHAM, A. (1992) *Lay Theories: Everyday Understanding of Problems in the Social Sciences*. Oxford: Pergamon Press.

GIFI, A. (1990) *Nonlinear Multivariate Analysis*. Chichester: John Wiley.

GLADWIN, C. H. (1989) *Ethnographic Decision Tree Modelling*. Newbury Park, CA: Sage.

GOLDBERG, D. & HUXLEY, P. (1980) *Mental Illness in the Community: The Pathway to Psychiatric Care*. London: Tavistock.

GREENACRE, M. (1992) Correspondence analysis in medical research. *Statistical Methods in Medical Research*, **1**, 97–117.

HELMAN, C. G. (1990) *Culture, Health and Illness* (2nd edn). Oxford: Butterworth-Heinemann.

KAPUR, R. L. (1979) The role of traditional healers in mental health care in rural India. *Social Science and Medicine*, **13B**, 27–31.

KIRMAYER, L. J. (1989) Cultural variations in the response of psychiatric disorders and emotional distress. *Social Science and Medicine*, **29**, 327–339.

—— (1991) The place of culture in psychiatric nosology: Taijin Kyofusho and DSM–III–R. *Journal of Nervous and Mental Diseases*, **179**, 19–28.

KLEINMAN, A. (1977) Depression, somatization and the 'new cross-cultural psychiatry'. *Social Science and Medicine*, **11**, 3–10.

LEFF, J. (1981) *Psychiatry Around the Globe: a Transcultural View*. New York: Marcel Dekker.

LITTLEWOOD, R. (1986) Russian dolls and Chinese boxes: an anthropological approach to the implicit models of comparative psychiatry. In *Transcultural Psychiatry* (ed. J. L. Cox). London: Croom Helm.

—— & LIPSEDGE, M. (1986) The 'culture-bound syndromes' of the dominant culture: culture, psychopathology and biomedicine. In *Transcultural Psychiatry* (ed. J. L. Cox). London: Croom Helm.

RACK, P. (1982) *Race, Culture and Mental Disorder*. London: Tavistock.

RICHARDSON, S. A., DOHRENWEND, B. S. & KLEIN, D. (1965) *Interviewing: Its Forms and Functions*. New York: Basic Books.

ROGLER, L. H. & CORTES, D. E. (1993) Help-seeking pathways: a unifying concept in mental health care. *American Journal of Psychiatry*, **150**, 554–561.

SENSKY, T. (1990) Patients' reactions to illness: cognitive factors determine responses and are amenable to treatment. *British Medical Journal*, **300**, 622–623.

SPSS (1990) *SPSS Categories*. Chicago: SPSS Inc.

SPRADLEY, J. P. (1979) *The Ethnographic Interview*. New York: Holt, Rinehart, and Winston.

—— (1980) *Participant Observation*. New York: Holt, Rinehart, and Winston.

ZOLA, I. K. (1966) Culture and symptoms: an analysis of patients' presenting complaints. *American Sociology Review*, **31**, 615–630.

Index

Compiled by LINDA ENGLISH